Inside God's Shed

Memoirs of an Intensive Care specialist

Lindsay I. G. Worthley

AM, MB BS, FRACP, FANZCA, FCICM

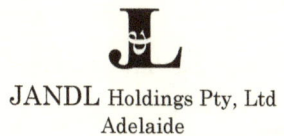

JANDL Holdings Pty, Ltd
Adelaide

Disclaimer
The opinions, comments and treatments outlined in individual cases do not indicate a recommendation for all or any such cases. Readers should not act on the basis of any matter in this publication without considering (and if appropriate, taking) professional advice with due regard to their own particular state and circumstances. The author and publisher expressly disclaim all and any liability to any person, whether a purchaser of this publication or not, in respect of anything and of the consequences of anything done or omitted to be done by any such person in reliance, whether whole or partial, upon the whole or any part of the contents of this publication.

Published in 2014 by
JANDL Holdings, Pty, Ltd
22 William St, Hawthorn
SOUTH AUSTRALIA 5062

Email: lindsaywrty@gmail.com

ISBN 978-0-9924306-0-3

©2014 JANDL Holdings Pty, Ltd
All rights reserved.
Requests to reproduce original material should be addressed to the publisher.

Printed and Bound in Australia

Contents

Preface vii

Abbreviations and Glossary ix

Introduction 1

Section 1 Clinical practice
What are intensive care units? 3
"The surgeon is pleased with the operation" 5
"So we think it's all over" 9
"Where's ol' knacker bags?" 12
"Do you think there is a God, doctor?" 14
"Bill's taking me home" 19
"But when I see him I get all confused" 23
Just when you thought that you could go home 26
Everything old is new again 29
At the coalface 32
The checklist is not something new 35
"Could we have a second opinion?" 39
Peanuts, pain, purgatory and persistence – at a price 44
If you tread on another intensivist's shoes – do it softly 51
Shhh! I think it's the patient 54
Please read the fine print 57
God heals and the doctor takes the fee 61
Protocols without thought are dangerous 65
"I'll be there in a minute" 68
Should the replacement of acute blood loss with non-red blood cell solutions in the elderly be called resuscitation or embalming? 71
"Mr. Smith would want to have the operation" 79
Spare me the pain 82
Cardiac arrest teams, medical emergency teams and rapid-response teams. Are we going backwards? 85

" . . . are you happy about that?"	91
The power of magic	94
Conventional medicine, complementary medicine and alternative medicine, or should they just be called medicine and unproven beliefs?	97
Bedside peer review: standards, judgment and sweet charity	105
"Do you wish your husband to be resuscitated?"	108
Quality control, risk and adverse events in the intensive care unit	110
"Oh . . . look at this"	118

Section 2. On death and dying

" . . . . and needs to be admitted to the ICU"	121
"While we often manage dying patients, dying is not an indication for admission to an ICU"	125
The dying patient	129
Right to die, withdrawal of therapy and the ICU as a medical purgatory	132
Critical care medicine and its cost	138

Section 3. Teaching and research

"I touch the future. I teach"	141
Cognitive development of the intensivist	144
Are intensive care units self-sustaining?	147
"If you knew 20 years ago what ICU medicine would be like today, do you think that you would still choose to be an intensivist?"	151
The ideal intensive care unit: open, closed or somewhere between?	154
The pro – con debate: educational, or just another blood sport?	158
Intravenous albumin: a waste of health dollars?	160
Naked in the electronic age	167
"We have a unique opportunity to offer you the newest treatment for . . . ."	171

The scientific journal: editorial freedom, freedom of
    expression and the pursuit of truth   174
"But . . . ?"   178

Section 4. Drug companies
    Can a doctor enjoy a medical company's generosity without
        prescribing its products?   180
    The Lancet is my hero; I shall not want   185
    Are drug companies using or abusing science?   187

Section 5. Reflections
    Do public hospital CEO's have a sense of humour?   193
    Return to my *Alma Mater*   197
    On reflection   200

Acknowledgements   205

About the Author   207

Index   209

Preface

I served as an Intensive Care specialist (Intensivist) for almost 40 years at five South Australian intensive care units, initially working at the Royal Adelaide Hospital intensive care unit (ICU), then at the Flinders Medical Centre ICU and also at three of Adelaide's private hospital ICUs. I retired from full time clinical practice and apart from some teaching and research sessions, most of my time now is spent with my dear wife, our three sons, and eight grandchildren. My moniker 'Tub' was given to me as a tease during my grade four year at St. Leonard's primary school, where I was perhaps as wide as I was tall. I have always accepted it as a term of endearment.

During my professional life I published many scientific articles and wrote several books on intensive care medicine. I was the editor of the Australasian intensive care medical journal *Critical Care and Resuscitation* (Crit Care Resusc) from 1999 to 2005. In this journal I published numerous human-interest stories as 'occasional essays', 'point of view' articles and editorials, highlighting some of the day-to-day issues that intensive care (critical care) specialists faced. As these stories appeared to resonate with many health care workers, I have decided to republish some of the articles, in modified form, along with the remaining untold essays, to complete my portrait of a general intensive care unit.

While the memoir will be of interest to the general reader, as it breaks down many of the medical stereotypes found in novels and TV shows, the text is predominantly that which will be familiar to health care professionals (i.e. doctors, nurses and paramedics). Nevertheless, to help the general reader, I have provided an 'Abbreviations and Glossary list' (see page ix – x) and have included a key to many of the acronyms used within each story. However, to give an explanation of each medical term or to sanitize the stories in a way to make them completely understandable to all, I believe would have ruined the spirit of the tome.

The stories in this book are true encounters, although many of the names have been either changed, or are not included to protect the grace and dignity of those involved. Those who are identified are already known and their stories are on public record. In looking back I trust that I have reflected with honesty, humanity and humour, and given a useful insight into the workings of major intensive care units.

L. I. G. Worthley
February 2014

Abbreviations and Glossary

A&E	Accident and Emergency
Actrapid®	recombinant human insulin
ALT	alanine aminotransferase
	(the blood level of ALT is high in liver damage)
Ambu™ bag	a hand operated breathing bag
ANZICS	Australian and New Zealand Intensive Care Society
AST	aspartate aminotransferase
	(the blood level of AST is high in liver damage)
BE	base excess
	(a measurement of alkalinity and acidity capacity in blood)
Bradycardia	slow pulse rate
CAM	complementary and alternative medical therapies
CPR	cardiopulmonary resuscitation
CRP	C-reactive protein
	(high with inflammation)
Cyanosed	bluish discolouration of skin, lips and fingernails
CV	curriculum vitae
CVC	central venous catheter
DDAVP®	1-deamino-8-A-arginine vasopressin
	(an i.v. dose increases plasma levels of a blood coagulant factor)
DT's	delirium tremens
EACA	epsilon aminocaproic acid
ECG	electrocardiograph
ECM	external cardiac massage
Gelofusine®	an artificial plasma substitute
GTN	glyceryl trinitrate
Hartmann's solution	a compound saline solution for intravenous use
HBV	hepatitis B virus
HCV	hepatitis C virus
HDU	high dependency unit
HIV	human immunodeficiency virus
Hypoalbuminaemia	low blood albumin level
Hypoinsulinaemia	low blood insulin level

Hypokalaemia	low blood potassium level
Hypotension	low blood pressure
Hypovolaemia	low blood volume
Hypoxic	low blood oxygen level
IABP	intra-aortic balloon pump
ICP	intracranial pressure
ICU	intensive care unit
INR	international normalised ratio (measures coagulability of blood)
Intensivist	Intensive Care specialist
i.v.	intravenous
Inotropic agents	agents that enhance cardiac contractility
Kyphoscoliosis	abnormal curvature of the spine
LD	lactic acid dehydrogenase (the blood level of LD is high in liver damage)
Marlex®	a plastic mesh used to reinforce a body defect (e.g. to cover a hernia)
MET	medical emergency team
NFR	not for resuscitation
$PaCO_2$	partial pressure of carbon dioxide in arterial blood
PaO_2	partial pressure of oxygen in arterial blood
PaOP	pulmonary artery occlusion pressure (high in heart failure e.g. > 18 mmHg)
Percutaneous	directly through skin
Pyrexia	elevated body temperature
RAH	Royal Adelaide Hospital
RBC	red blood cells
RCT	randomised controlled trial
SNP	sodium nitroprusside (an intravenous agent used to reduce blood pressure)
ST	part of an ECG trace that reflects cardiac injury
Swan Ganz catheter	right heart flotation catheter (used to measure intracardiac pressure and cardiac output)
Tachycardia	fast pulse rate
VF	ventricular fibrillation
VT	ventricular tachycardia

Introduction

"If I had my life to live over again, I would have made a rule to read some poetry and listen to some music at least once a week; for perhaps the parts of my brain now atrophied would have thus been kept active through use. The loss of these tastes is a loss of happiness, and may possibly be injurious to the intellect, and more probably to the moral character, by enfeebling the emotional part of our nature."
Charles Darwin

"Mum he's touching me!" I stopped the car. My wife got into the back seat and positioned herself between our two eldest boys.

"Muuuuum . . . he's looking at me!"

I looked through the rear vision mirror to see my youngest son Daniel, being nursed by my wife. He was smiling, oblivious to the bubble of mucus protruding in and out of his nostril (he's now a gastroenterologist). On my wife's right side was my eldest son Stephen (now a cardiologist), protesting that my middle son Matthew (also a cardiologist), on her left side was 'looking' at him. Matthew was staring out the window trying to look as if he was an innocent bystander.

As I was remembering these early years, approximately 35 years later, Matthew opened my office door and asked me to help him with a cardioversion for one of his patients. We both worked at the same private hospital, and the intensive care specialist on call – me on this occasion – often provided the anaesthetic for cardioversions required by the visiting cardiologist – him on this occasion.

"Sure, mate" I said, and wandered down the hallway chatting idly about friends who had been staying with us for the last few days. I had approximately one year left before I retired: 57 weeks to be exact. I was enjoying my clinical practice, unencumbered by teaching, research and administrative duties, as I had retired from my public intensive care practice more than two years previously.

1

L. I. G. Worthley

Interestingly, as I aged I began to think more about my patients: their diagnoses, ongoing management and likely prognoses. At night I would try to get to sleep by performing a mental intensive care unit ward round, and if awoken by someone requesting me to see a critically ill patient, I needed to listen to an album by the 70's 'soft rock' group 'Bread' while driving in, to allow me to calmly consider the patient's problem. I was finding it more and more difficult to psychologically escape the unit. My retirement was probably necessary for my well-being.

Now, six years after performing the anaesthetic for Matthew's patient and five years into my retirement, I have decided to publish a number of stories about my professional life. I trust that most of these stories have held the test of time and that from this distance I can see a little clearer.

Section 1. Clinical practice

What are intensive care units?

"ICUs are areas where extraordinary accomplishments and extraordinary waste live side by side, and often where no serious attempt is made to draw a line between the two."
G.C. Carlon[1]

The intensive care unit (ICU) is a dedicated hospital area designed for the management of patients with sudden, or potentially sudden, and reversible life-threatening conditions. It is the central hub of a major hospital and contains specialised monitoring devices including machines to measure cardiac rhythm, blood pressure, blood gas and blood biochemistry; as well as life support equipment that include defibrillators, mechanical ventilators, circulatory pumps and dialysers – to support a failing heart, lungs or kidneys. It is staffed by medical and nursing specialists who are trained and skilled in diagnosing and treating immediate life-threatening conditions.

It is commonly believed that intensive care medicine, as a specialty, began with the 1952-1953 Danish poliomyelitis epidemic, where Bjørn Ibsen and Henry Lassen at Copenhagen's Blegdam Hospital reported a reduction in mortality from 87% to 25% in more than 300 polio patients treated by prolonged mechanical positive pressure ventilation. They ventilated patients through a tracheotomy tube to maintain respiration (oxygen delivery and carbon dioxide removal) and protect the airway while the polio-induced respiratory muscle paralysis resolved.[2] Subsequently, an earlier paper by Albert Bower was discovered in an obscure medical journal, which reported a survival rate of 83.7% in 129 polio patients at the Los Angeles County General Hospital using long-term positive pressure ventilation.[3]

For the previous two decades, positive pressure ventilation tended to be restricted to operating rooms, whereas negative pressure tank

3

ventilators were used for prolonged mechanical ventilatory support. However, as severe polio caused both respiratory muscle and pharyngeal muscle paralysis, mortality was not reduced when negative pressure tank ventilators without a tracheostomy were used, as the patient would suffocate in their oral and respiratory secretions.

Following the success of positive pressure ventilation in the management of polio victims, intensive care units were created during the 1950's and 60's throughout Europe, the UK, USA and Australia. The specialty of intensive care medicine also developed with the formation of numerous intensive and critical care societies and colleges, which provided specialised training and accreditation in acute medical care.

Fundamentally, intensive care units provide critical support for vital organs while specific therapies – for example surgery, intravenous fluids, antibiotics, etc – allow enough time for the body's natural reparative processes to resolve the acute illness. William Knaus encapsulated this by saying "The best a good ICU care can accomplish is to reverse acute physiological abnormalities and buy time. If during this time, therapy works or the body mounts its own attack, the patient will live. If not, then all ICU care can achieve is delay".[4] While amazing results can be achieved when patients are managed in these units, distraught relatives and occasionally inexperienced practitioners may have unrealistic expectations. The patient, at best, can only be returned to their prior condition; the chronic underlying illnesses are rarely, if ever, corrected by ICU treatment.

REFERENCES
1. Carlon GC. Just say no. Crit Care Med 1989;17:106-107.
2. Trubuhovich RV. In the beginning. The 1952-1953 Danish epidemic of poliomyelitis and Bjørn Ibsen. Crit Care Resusc 2003;5:227-230.
3. Trubuhovich RV. On the very first, successful, long-term, large scale use of IPPV. Albert Bower and V Ray Bennett: Los Angeles, 1948-1949. Crit Care Resusc 2007;9:91-100.
4. Knaus WA. Changing the cause of death. JAMA 1983;249:1059-1060.

"The surgeon is pleased with the operation"

"My advice to you concerning applause is this; enjoy it but never quite believe it."
Robert Montgomery

I was on duty at the private hospital ICU and awaiting the arrival of the third cardiac surgical patient planned for the day. It was late on Friday night and the patient had already been in theatre for three hours. The first indication of any activity came when the theatre nurse entered the unit requesting an intra-aortic balloon pump (IABP) to help disconnect the patient from cardiopulmonary bypass without causing a severe reduction in blood pressure. Apparently, the surgeon had attempted to take the patient 'off' bypass in theatre twice previously but without success.

When asked about the patient's condition, she rolled her eyes and said "A lot of swearing is going on."

"Terrific!" I thought, I knew the likely scenario. The patient would be returned to the ICU on a large dose of adrenaline, with a temporary pacemaker, blood would be welling from all chest drains and the balloon pump would be 'ticking away' on full augmentation.

I phoned my wife to tell her the news. "I'll probably be home some time after midnight, sweetie."

After another 45 minutes, the doors of the ICU suddenly opened and the patient was brought in with a constant beeping of the cardiac monitor, clanking of drainage bottles and hiss of oxygen. After the bed was correctly positioned, I wandered over to the patient and watched the nursing staff go into automatic mode: shift the mechanical ventilator into place, help the anaesthetist connect the anaesthetic circuit to the ventilator, disconnect the cardiac leads from the defibrillator and replace them with the ICU monitoring leads, reconnect the chest drain suctioning system and tidy the bed.

"Not a pretty sight," the anaesthetist said as he pulled his gloves off. "The adrenaline is on 20 micrograms per minute with occasional boluses to keep the mean arterial pressure above 60 mmHg, and that's with full balloon augmentation. Oh, by the way," he added, "the pacemaker sometimes doesn't capture, leaving an underlying nodal rate of about 30 beats a minute with bursts of VT which usually revert spontaneously – although we had to shock him twice for VF before we left theatre."

"Terrific. The patient's good then?" I said with a heavy dose of sarcasm.

"Hmm . . ." he smirked, half closing his eyes "have fun!" He left carrying the portable oxygen cylinder, defibrillator, and the latest 'Home & Garden' journal under his arm.

The surgeon arrived 5 minutes later. "He's got diabetic coronary vessels – small, deep in fat, impossible to get at. I had to put five grafts in to try and resurrect some blood supply to a totally wrecked left ventricle" he grumbled.

"Uh," I said pumping in the third pint of blood, adding "he seems a little 'wet', so we are also giving him platelets, fresh frozen plasma and some DDAVP®. What was he like when you closed him?"

"He wasn't too bad. What about trying some EACA?" the surgeon replied.

"Sure" I said, although I believed that EACA administration would just be tinkering at the edges as the chest drain loss suggested a surgical bleeding problem. "We will see what we can do."

He turned and left saying that he should be home in 20 minutes, and for us to let him know if there was any change.

The ICU charge nurse hurried in and said that she had just been talking to the relatives in the waiting room and that they wished to see the patient.

"Could you please usher them into my office. I will have a chat to them first before they come in and see him," I replied, now pumping in the fourth unit of blood.

Thankfully, for the next ten minutes, the patient appeared to be relatively stable, so I thought that I would take the opportunity to talk to the family.

Inside God's Shed

His wife and two daughters were sitting nervously in my room around the conference table. They looked intently at me as I walked in to join them. "How is he, doctor?" the wife asked.

"Well . . . " I said, "perhaps I will begin after you have filled me in with what you already know, so that I don't have to travel over old ground again." I pulled my desk chair around so that I could sit with them at the table.

"Well doctor, the surgeon said that he was pleased with the operation, and that apart from a few problems, he should make a good recovery – although he did say that he was still critically ill at the moment and needed to get over the long anaesthetic. He said that the next 6 to 12 hours would be crucial."

Pleased with the operation! Make a good recovery! But why should I be surprised? I don't think that I have ever heard a surgeon talk to a patient about his or her operation and say that they weren't "pleased with the operation." However, in this case, the patient was in ICU and dying, and perhaps, as far as the family could tell, if he did die, the ICU specialist (i.e. me) would be largely responsible.

As with so many conversations with relatives of patients who are critically ill and being managed in the ICU, a realistic description of the situation without telling them to lose all hope is required. Such statements as "we will be doing everything possible" and "please be patient" and "he will be in no pain" and "at least he has not deteriorated" are often used to calm frayed nerves, particularly when the ICU episode drags on for days.

Thankfully, the patient did survive, after: returning to theatre 4 hours later to treat the surgical bleeding problem (none was said to be found, yet the blood loss became a trickle immediately afterwards), 18 units of blood, 4 packs of fresh frozen plasma, 2 packs of platelets and 7 days on the IABP, to be discharged from the ICU after two weeks.

He returned to the ICU ten days later in a wheel chair pushed by his beaming wife. He had just seen the surgeon who was pleased, and probably relieved, at the final outcome. His wife wished to thank all the medical and nursing staff involved. He appeared to be slightly confused while shaking the hands of all and sundry, with porters and cleaning staff joining in. He did not remember being in the ICU at all, and certainly did not remember me, although he did remember the ICU nurse who looked after him just before he was discharged from the unit – he said she was an angel and gave her a large box of assorted sweets as a gratuity.

Such is life in the ICU. If you wish to be remembered by an eternally grateful patient, after spending hours of your mental and physical energy attempting to avert an impending death, don't become an intensivist.

" So we think it's all over"

"Never give in. Never give in. Never, never, never, never – in nothing, great or small, large or petty – never give in."
  Winston Churchill

I was wandering through the Accident and Emergency (A&E) department one Monday evening when I came across Jenny, our ICU registrar, and David, the A&E consultant, doing cardiopulmonary resuscitation (CPR) on a patient.
"What's happening Jenny?" I asked.
"Oh, a young lad was found unconscious in one of the city laneways and was brought in pulseless. We are just about to give up, as we are unable to get him out of a rhythm that varies between slow VF and asystole. Adrenaline doesn't work, and amiodarone and lignocaine produce asystole. We think it's all over."
"Can I have a look?" I said reaching for the Ambu™ bag.
"Sure" said Jenny, who gave me the bag, took her gloves off and sat down to record the events.
"Have you taken any blood?" I said, not wishing to impose too much into the treatment of the cardiac arrest.
"No," said Jenny. David, who was still performing external cardiac massage, suddenly spoke. "Didn't think it was any use as the patient would be acidotic and hypoxic so we decided to just treat him empirically."
"Sure, Dave, but the patient seems to have a strange sweet smell about him."
"Yeah, apparently some vodka the lad took as well as his heroin," said David who by now was starting to drip sweat from his chin.
"But vodka doesn't smell. Do you have any other history – from his parents, ambulance driver or anybody else?" I asked.
"Nup – John Doe" said Jenny who continued writing.
I quietly wondered whether the CPR team had misread the boy's problem by diagnosing him as a heroin overdose, when perhaps he

9

may have been a diabetic with ketoacidosis, with acetone giving him his 'sweet smell', and severe hyperkalaemia causing his resistant cardiac rhythm.

"Well, that's it!" said David who suddenly stopped external cardiac massage, "we've been going now for more than 45 minutes."

"But his pupils are still small," I said. "What about a few more minutes?"

"OK" he said, and beckoned to one of the nurses.

"You have a go. See how long you can do ECM without getting tired." The nurse began ECM while I continued ventilating the patient.

"Jenny," I said, "has the patient had any calcium chloride?"

"Not recommended in the standard protocol," David chimed in.

"I know that," I said "but I think this boy may have hyperkalaemia, so a burst of calcium before we give up on him may be worth a try."

"Go your hardest" was his reply. He obviously felt that any further treatment would be futile so he walked out, leaving Jenny, myself, and the nurse to continue.

"Jenny, can you get me a blood gas syringe and 10 mL of calcium chloride. I reckon the boy has severe diabetic ketoacidosis with hyperkalaemia and that's why he's resistant to standard CPR treatment."

A blood gas was taken from his femoral artery and 10 mL of 10% calcium chloride was given as an intravenous bolus. Suddenly, sinus rhythm appeared on the ECG monitor.

"I can feel a pulse!" said Jenny "What a gun! Wait till I tell David."

"Don't bother," I said. "We need to sedate the lad before he pulls the endotracheal tube out, and get him up to the ICU . . . fast!"

The boy had an arterial blood glucose of 55 mmol/L (normally 3 – 6 mmol/L), pH of 6.9 (normally 7.35 – 7.45), potassium 8.8 mmol/L (normally 3.1 – 4.2 mmol/L) and bicarbonate of 1 mmol/L (normally 22 – 31 mmol/L). We treated him with an insulin infusion and 3 litres of intravenous fluid during the first 12 hours. He was extubated 18 hours after his cardiac arrest and amazingly appeared to be alert, orientated, and apart from a tender chest, in no discomfort. He was subsequently found to be a type 1 diabetic who normally lived in Melbourne but went to Adelaide for the Easter weekend. As his friends were unaware of his diabetes, he decided not to take his insulin. Early on Monday night, after a day of feeling unwell and intermittently vomiting, he left his apartment and was found unconscious in a side street. He was admitted to the RAH with a provisional diagnosis of 'drug overdose.'

He was discharged from the Royal Adelaide Hospital after 5 days, with no neurological defect and back onto his normal insulin dose.

Adult intensive care units commonly treat octogenarian patients who have many chronic illnesses as well as their acute, and hopefully reversible, critical illness. They either respond very slowly and usually incompletely, or not at all. To have a patient who is young and who responds so dramatically and completely, is very gratifying.

"Where's ol' knacker bags?"

"If you get to thinking you're a person of some influence, try ordering somebody else's dog around."
Will Rogers

The insertion of a central venous catheter (CVC) is often performed under local anaesthesia. However patients who require intravenous access often, and over a prolonged period, (e.g. leukaemic patients) soon develop needle phobia, and need deep sedation or even general anaesthesia for the procedure. One such patient was referred to me with the request "could he be 'put under' while the CVC line is inserted, because one week ago he had a very painful experience when a CVC insertion was attempted unsuccessfully at one of the public hospitals." He was admitted to the private hospital so that an 'expert' could be called in to deal with the problem, and as it was my rostered week on at the private hospital's intensive care unit, I was the default 'expert.'

I introduced myself to the patient and said that we would first ultrasound his neck to review the venous anatomy as the previous attempt may have failed due to a vascular abnormality. This was performed and demonstrated large upper torso veins with normal anatomical positioning. I returned to the patient and stated that the veins did not pose any particular difficulty for central venous access, and that I would give him some 'deep sedation' to alleviate his anxiety and any pain during the procedure.

After preparing my tray and positioning the patient, I prepared the skin site and readied myself at the bedside. I gave him an initial 3 mg of midazolam intravenously followed 1 minute later by a further 2 mg. While he was placid after the initial intravenous drugs, he was still very much awake, so I gave him some intravenous propofol, to a total of 7 mL over 1 to 2 minutes, which finally made his eyes close. I then began to infiltrate the skin site overlying the right subclavian vein with 1% lignocaine, during which the patient mumbled and winced slightly.

Inside God's Shed

I inserted the Seldinger wire into the right subclavian vein and then inserted the catheter over the wire, secured the catheter to the skin with a stitch and dressed the site with a clear bandage. Two minutes later, while the catheter position was being confirmed with a chest X-ray, the patient began to awake up.

"When will you get underway Doc?" the patient mumbled.

"It's already done," I said.

"Really?" he asked, now opening his eyes wide and slowly looking around to find the catheter firmly plastered to his right shoulder. He was amazed. The procedure had already been performed while he was oblivious to anything being done.

As it is with certain sedative agents, particularly during the first few minutes of the arousal, the patient often awakens in a euphoric state, which happened with this patient. He loudly declared that his doctor was a 'real expert', 'the best in the world', 'he was brilliant' and 'I didn't even feel a thing.'

While I knew that the sedative agents had made him delusional, I milked the occasion to all the hapless nursing and medical staff who were present.

"Hear the man," I said – "what else can I say?" Nevertheless, just before he was sent back to the ward he stated drowsily to the attending nurse, "Where's old knacker bags?"

"Who?" she replied.

"You know, ol' knacker bags - the chubby little doctor with the bulgy eyes. The one who inserted the catheter. I want to thank him again."

The nursing staff lined up, maybe 3 to 4 deep, all jostling to relate this story to me.

"Do you think there is a God, doctor?"

"We are guests in our patients' lives."
Donald Berwick

As well as managing patients who have an acute life-threatening illness in the intensive care unit, part of the intensivist's career may involve managing patients requiring prolonged life support (e.g. intravenous nutrition) at home.

A normal adult human will adapt to periods of starvation for up to 30 days without any demonstrable adverse effects. Periods of starvation in excess of this will lead to nutritional depletion causing respiratory muscle weakness, diminished immune defence and poor wound healing, with death occurring after 60 days.[1] In disease, and in malnourished states, starvation is poorly tolerated and a correlation often exists between the degree of starvation and the patient's outcome. Intravenous (parenteral) nutrition to treat malnourished patients was first reported in 1968 by Stanley Dudrick *et al.*[2] The fluids were administered through a central venous catheter and contained electrolytes, concentrated glucose, amino acids and vitamins. Subsequent solutions included lipids and trace elements. As intensivists were skilled in inserting central venous catheters in patients who had difficult peripheral venous access, they were often asked to provide the same service for patients who needed parenteral nutrition. Intensivists would also periodically extend their services to manage these patients at home. The solutions were infused throughout the night using a pump. The patient would disconnect him or herself in the morning, and would be unencumbered and ambulant throughout the day.

Throughout my career, I managed 34 home parenteral nutrition patients and often spent many hours talking to them about a range of topics. Three patients left me with enduring memories.

Inside God's Shed

"Do you think there is a God, doctor?" was a question from one home parenteral nutrition patient who had terminal gastric cancer. She had undergone surgery, chemotherapy and even tried alternative medical therapies in an attempt to manage her malignant growth. Ultimately, due to gastric outlet obstruction, she began to vomit, and required parenteral nutrition to sustain her during her final months. She refused to have a tube inserted either directly through her abdomen, or through her nose, to remove the gastric fluid, or to have a tube inserted into her small intestine to infuse food directly into her bowel, as she felt that these would limit her mobility and continually remind her of her illness. A nightly infusion of intravenous nutrition and a morning and evening vomit appeared to her as the better option. Apart from moderate weakness requiring a walking stick for assistance, she complained of no pain nor discomfort and had a remarkable zest for life. She knew the cancer was incurable but wished to live with it, rather than spend her last few days thinking about dying from it.

"An omnipotent God: well what do you think?" I would say.

She would continue: "Do you think there is an after-life?" and without waiting for an answer, "do religions appeal to people because they promise an eternal after-life?"

I often just smiled and held her hand. We had had numerous exchanges like this, although I often felt that she just wanted me to listen rather than talk, as she would tend to resolve her own uncertainties to her satisfaction, and ultimately find peace.

We discussed – consciousness: "have you thought about what it is to be you or me?" – reincarnation: "why should my conscious state re-emerge, even after millions of years?" – evolution: "if we have evolved over millions of years we must still be evolving. What will we be like in 100,000 or a million of years from now?" – even the concept of time: "will we will ever reverse time?"

I often visited her on my 'free' Wednesday afternoons. It was summer and the sun would send shards of light through her bedroom window. Her husband and son were in the next room, not necessarily ignoring us, but unwilling to confront the reality of a wife and mother who was dying and receiving a strange form of palliation from me. Yet in her room I was allowed to enter a space where her ego had disappeared. We talked freely about anything. It was a remarkable experience.

She died from pneumonia three months later.

"If Jesus was the Son of God and Man, why do we need to believe in a virgin birth? Surely it would be more relevant to humanity if it were not," was one of the many provocations a retired Uniting Church minister, a man who was probably born before his time, would level at me. His wife, whom I had treated with parenteral nutrition due to malnutrition caused by an extensive radiation enteritis, had 'crossed the river' many years ago. However, I kept in contact with this dear man and would attempt to visit him every month. He believed that Christianity was attracting fundamentalists who held beliefs that were not only unappealing to the younger generation, but were utterly wrong and would often boom, "The church must change or die!"

He was deeply interested in literature. If I entered his room at the retirement village while he was reading, he would promptly recite a line or two.

"Come on at a footpace! D'ye mind me? And if you've got holsters to that saddle o' yourn, don't let me see your hand go nigh 'em. For I'm a devil at a quick mistake, and when I make one it takes the form of lead. So now let's look at you!"

"What do you think of that?" he would ask.

"Terrific," I would enthuse.

"Dickens," he would proclaim.

He died aged 92. It would be nice to meet him again in the hereafter. However, while my great grandfather was a Methodist minister, and my mother went to church each Sunday night, I guess I am more like my father who would say politely, when asked about his belief in God and an after-life, that he wasn't really an atheist, he was an agnostic. I remember as a young boy, my sister and I would ask him,

"Dad, why don't you go to church with mum?"

He would reply with a twinkle in his eye. "Church is for sinners."

Inside God's Shed

A Spanish lady developed frequent episodes of bowel obstruction following an appendicectomy performed when she was a teenager. The obstructive episodes were treated surgically with numerous bowel resections, and ultimately she was referred to me at the Royal Adelaide Hospital to manage her severe malnutrition with parenteral nutrition. At this stage, she had one large, and two small enteric fistulas. The large fistula would intermittently close at skin level and develop a blind fistula, largely because the distal bowel was partially obstructed. When this occurred, an abdominal abscess would form, her surgeon would refer her to the radiology department and a radiologist would drain the abscess percutaneously. The distal bowel obstruction would remain.

Following each episode, the fistula drained for a few weeks, closed, developed into a blind fistula, an abscess would form and require drainage again. When I transferred to the Flinders Medical Centre, I continued her management. The lady, as expected, developed her fistula closure and subsequent abdominal abscess. I asked her if she wanted to see her surgeon again who would arrange for the abscess to be drained.

"Please don't send me to that butcher. Could I see someone else here?" she pleaded.

"Sure," I said making no indication one way or another of my thoughts – even though I felt she probably should have had a second opinion some time ago, and probably had a different surgeon managing her case.

She saw another surgeon who operated and corrected her distal bowel obstruction, closed her fistulas and drained the abdominal abscesses. Thereafter, she had no further surgical abdominal problems. Unfortunately, by this time, she had less than the necessary length of small bowel to allow her to manage her nutrition by mouth. Nevertheless, she was delighted with the surgical result and did not mind remaining on her parenteral nutrition therapy.

This episode left me with many questions.

What should one do if you believe a clinician is incompetent, particularly when they are involved with one of the patients under your care? Had I been wrong to ignore my patient's surgical problems? When healthcare staff such as nurse Toni Hoffman and Dr. Peter

Miach started to whistleblow at Bundaberg Base Hospital, Queensland, concerning Dr. Jayant Patel's alleged negligent medical practice, they were threatened with measures to compel their silence.[3] Dr. Patel was subsequently found guilty of three counts of manslaughter and one count of grievous bodily harm – although the High Court upheld his appeal and ordered a re-trial for one of the manslaughter charges.[4] The jury acquitted Dr. Patel and the remaining charges were later dropped in exchange for Patel pleading guilty to two counts related to him dishonestly gaining registration and two counts related to dishonestly gaining employment in Queensland. He was sentenced to a two year suspended sentence for those fraud charges.[5]

While whistleblowing may be necessary for patient safety, it is hazardous for the whistleblower.

REFERENCES
1. Korcok M. Hunger strikers may have died of fat, not protein, loss. JAMA 1981;246:1878-1879.
2. Dudrick SJ, Wilmore DW, Vars HM, Rhoads JE. Long-term total parenteral nutrition with growth, development and positive nitrogen balance. Surgery 1968;64:134-142.
3. Morris T. Bundaberg butcher not the only culprit. http://www.theaustralian.com.au/news/nation/bundaberg-butcher-not-the-only-culprit/story-e6frg6nf-1225885901700 (accessed February 2012).
4. High Court orders Patel retrial after 'miscarriage of justice'. www.abc.net.au/ news/2012-08-24/patel-wins-high-court-appeal/4220380 (accessed August 2012).
5. Norton F, Rawlins J. Former Bundaberg-based doctor Jayant Patel sentenced over fraud charges. http://www.abc.net.au/news/2013-11-21/jayant-patel-sentenced-over-fraud-charges/5107314 (accessed November 2013).

"Bill's taking me home"

"a lie is useless to the gods, and useful only as a medicine to men."
Plato

"Captain, captain, where's the captain?" his head swung wildly from one side to the other. I had just walked through the door of an isolation bay in response to a ward medical emergency team (MET) call concerning a patient who was having an acute psychotic episode.

"Bill, Bill!" he barked as he turned his head sharply left and looked at the door. I looked back and saw no one.

The nurse tried to calm him "Mr. Smith, you are in hospital and your brother is *not* coming in."

"Bill, Bill!" he screamed, as he arched his back.

The nurse looked exasperated as she tried reasoning with the patient and turned to me, "Could you please help? We are struggling to keep Mr. Smith in bed. He has pulled his drip out and he wants to go home. We phoned his brother but he does *not* want to talk to him and said he won't be coming in."

I looked at the patient who was struggling against four beefy orderlies. He was sweating, wide-eyed and in no mood for rational conversation.

"What's he in hospital for?" I asked.

The nurse explained that Mr. Reginald Smith was a 68 year old alcoholic who had suddenly became severely agitated 3 days after an operative insertion of an Austin Moore prosthesis for his fractured neck of femur. He had been quiet for most of the morning but refused his breakfast or any medications, as he believed that the nursing staff were trying to poison him.

"He's having a bad case of DT's," I said. "Where's the orthopaedic team?"

"They're all in theatre. They told me to dial a MET call when I told them about Mr. Smith."

"Nothing unusual there," I thought. "Does he have any recent blood results?"

She showed me the biochemical and haematological results from the morning's venesection round which surprised me somewhat as orthopaedic wards tend to ignore blood tests.

Apart from a mild anaemia (haemoglobin 101 g/L), slight hypokalaemia (potassium 3.1 mmol/L), and elevation of the alkaline phosphatase (220 IU/L) the glucose, sodium and remaining liver function tests were within normal limits. I turned to the nurse,

"Could you get me 10 mg of Valium® and 100 mg of chlorpromazine in separate syringes please? Also, I'll need a 20 gauge i.v. cannula, some 'hep' saline in a 10 mL syringe, a bung and couple of alcohol swabs."

"He's already had 10 mg of Valium® i.v. twice," she said.

"Well… bring the syringe of chlorpromazine and have the Valium® on hand."

I then turned to the patient.

"Reg," I said.

"Yes, Mr. De Silver," he replied, as he spun his head around to look in my direction (I thought later, that my white gown in a sea of blue and black clothing worn by the nurse and orderlies may have made me appear 'silver' to a hallucinating man).

"What do you want?" I asked.

"I wanna get out – help me, help me!" and once again he tried to lift himself up. The orderlies checked his movements.

"Where're you going?" I asked.

"Home! Bill's taking me home – there he is… Bill, Bill!" he spun his head around and looked at the doorway. Again, no one was there.

"Bill's coming back in a minute, Reg. He's just gone for a piss. He'll be back in a minute," I said.

He looked up at the orderlies holding his hands "Let go my hands!" He demanded. They remained silent.

The nurse arrived with a 20 gauge i.v. cannula, an interlink Luer lock bung, 5 mL syringe of heparinised saline and a 5 mL syringe with 100 mg of chlorpromazine. Reg was still writhing under the orderlies restraint and now believed that everyone was trying to kill him, howling,

"Help me, heeeelp me . . . . . somebody help me!"

I asked one of the orderlies to hold his right hand and arm firmly to allow me to insert the intravenous cannula.

"Reg," I said, "Bill is getting some help and is coming back to get you out of here, so we'll get you ready."

I quickly wiped the back of his hand with an alcohol swab and inserted the cannula into a large vein, causing blood to spurt out the end.

"Ow, what's that?" he demanded.

"Bill wanted an ID code on the back of your hand – to get you past the front door."

Reg wriggled as he looked around suspiciously. I capped the cannula and infused an intravenous bolus of 100 mg of chlorpromazine followed by 5 mL of heparin saline.

"Ow, ow, ow!" his cries soon became less frequent and less intense.

Just then the ward intern entered.

"Do you need a hand?"

"No – everything's under control. We've given Reg a large i.v. dose of 'chlorprom' so we will need to admit him to ICU" I said, and went to the sink to wash the blood from my hands.

"Can I have the sphygmo?" I said to the nurse, "and could you call the ICU ward and say that I am bringing a Mr. Reginald Smith back with me. And could they please set up for an arterial line!"

His BP was 110/50 mmHg. I turned to the intern and said, "don't ever use i.v. chlorpromazine, particularly in a shocked patient because it will cause a severe drop in blood pressure." He looked confused. "It's a vasodilator – an alpha adrenergic blocker – even in minute doses. I used it in Reg," I added, "because we needed to control his delirium rapidly. And in a vasodilated psychotic patient it has a minimal cardiovascular effect and a predominant tranquilising and soporific effect – particularly when Valium® has been used." He nodded and smiled, and realized that I had used it largely as an anaesthetic agent.

L. I. G. Worthley

"Let's get moving," I said hoping to have the orderlies, who by now had stopped holding Reg, help me move his bed and the resuscitation equipment to the ICU.

"Why did you ridicule him?" the nurse said suddenly. She obviously felt that I had in some way violated Reg.

"God spare me!" I thought.

"Nurse, I did not endeavour to make fun of him to entertain you and the orderlies. There was absolutely no point in attempting to reason with Mr. Smith. He's psychotic. To even get some semblance of cooperation, you have to enter his deluded world as a friend. To do anything else will just make him scream."

I turned to the orderlies, "let's get underway chaps!"

"But when I see him I get all confused"

*"I keep six honest serving-men
(They taught me all I knew);
Their names are What and Why and When
And How and Where and Who"*
    Rudyard Kipling

I had just finished explaining to the family of patient who had undergone a coronary artery bypass graft and was admitted to the ICU, what had happened, what we intended to do and what the likely outcome would be, when, in the process of ushering them out of my office, one of the relatives turned to me:

"Can I speak to you for a moment doctor?" It was the patient's sister-in law.

"Sure" I said. I invited her back, closed the door and asked her to sit down.

"Doctor, I know that this is not in your area, but I would value your advice. I have been diagnosed with lymphoma," she began.

"Oh, I am sorry to hear that," I replied.

She looked down and continued, saying that she had been referred to an oncology specialist and had seen him, now, three times.

"But when I see him, I get all confused. At our last meeting he finally told me I had a non-Hodgkin's lymphoma but it seemed like an afterthought. When I leave his office, I realize that I have not asked all the questions I need to. I feel rushed. I have been on the internet and what I read is frightening me."

She stopped for a moment and closed her eyes to compose herself. I lent over to hold her hand. She smiled and seemed to relax a little.

"Doctor, what I really wanted to ask is, should I see someone else?"

I knew the oncologist she had been referred to. He was an excellent practitioner – when gauged by the yardstick of keeping up with the latest treatment of various cancers and wanting support from every medical specialty for his patients. However he was a humourless character and could only converse on medical matters. He would often badger the intensive care specialist for a bed in ICU for one of his elderly septicaemic neutropaenic cancer patients, and was unwilling to reach a diagnosis of 'futility' or accept 'withdrawal of therapy' when such a point had been reached.

"I know your doctor well," I began, "and although he can be a little terse, he's an expert in his field and he does care for his patients in his own, perhaps unusual, way. I genuinely don't think that seeing someone else will help."

She shuffled a little with embarrassment.

"However I can understand how you must feel with this chap, with all those diplomas on the wall behind him. Nevertheless, you must remember you are the most important person in that room. Have your questions prepared on a piece of paper before you see him, and refer to them during your discussion."

"Would he be annoyed if I did that?" she said.

"Of course not, and if he appeared to be a little troubled, that's his bad luck," I replied and added, "I don't mind if you want to see me after seeing him. Perhaps I could interpret what he has said, and tell you the questions to ask him next time."

This arrangement worked well. And after the next consultation she said that she did not need to see me again as she had formed a firm and trusting relationship with her oncologist.

An illness, particularly a serious one, reduces the patient to a common denominator. They are frightened, dependent, confused and vulnerable. Clinicians who wish to provide their care, need to listen to them, observe them and think about them. There are no substitutes for these simple principles. When a patient enters the doctor's office they want reassurance. Are the symptoms benign? If not, is the diagnosis correct? If so, is the condition curable? If the condition is not curable the patient must feel that the doctor will be with them throughout their illness. Discussions should be honest, frank but never brutal, and hope should never be crushed.

The questions are always the same, and include:
- What do I have? (i.e. what is the diagnosis?)
- Could it be anything else? (i.e. is the diagnosis certain?)
- Do I need any more tests, and if so what are they?
- What will happen if I have no treatment? (i.e. what will be the course of the disease without treatment?)
- What is the treatment?
- What are the alternatives?
- What are the risks and benefits of each?
- What will the treatment do? (if multiple drugs are needed, what does each do?)
- What are the side effects of each drug and should I contact you if they develop?
- How long do I take the treatment?
- When are the beneficial effects expected to begin?
- Will it cure the disease, or just modify the symptoms?

I remember on one occasion, as a young trainee intensivist, I complained to a senior intensive care nurse about a terminal chronic respiratory failure patient who would continually question me about his management and then not adhere to my treatment. She just smiled and said, "Love your patients, Tub." My wife reminds me of this whenever I stray in my conversation with her about 'My day.'

Just when you thought that you could go home

"It is hard to teach new dogs old tricks."
Warren Buffett

There wasn't much to be excited about this week. Everything I did appeared to hinder rather than help the patients. Thank goodness it was the weekend. Finally, after a long and arduous Saturday ward round with an unenthusiastic registrar, I left the unit and was climbing into my car when suddenly my phone rang with a message to contact the 'on call' cardiologist.

"I've got a patient who needs to be admitted to the intensive care unit" he said. I remained silent.

"Are you still there?" he said after a few seconds.

"Yes," I said "I was waiting for you to tell me the story."

Apparently he had been managing an 80 year old man who had a one week history of increasing nausea and a four day history of intermittent vomiting, renal failure and jaundice. The patient had a past history of chronic heart failure that had been treated with captopril, frusemide and spironolactone. While a provisional diagnosis of hepatitis had been made, with no history of a recent exposure to hepatotoxins and negative tests for viral agents known to cause hepatitis, the cardiologist thought that the patient was 'septic' and that ongoing treatment with antibiotics and inotropic agents would be necessary.

"Admit him to the intensive care unit and I will see what we can do," I said, as I got out of my car and returned slowly to the unit.

When I saw the patient, he had cyanosis of ears, fingers and knees, a blood pressure of 140/75 mmHg, a weak pulse of 54 beats per minute and a temperature of 36.8°C. The chest X-ray revealed a large heart with no signs of pulmonary oedema. A blood biochemical profile performed that morning revealed a sodium concentration of 130 mmol/L, creatinine 0.53 µmol/L, alanine aminotransferase (ALT)

1104 U/L, aspartate aminotransferase (AST) 967 U/L, lactic acid dehydrogenase (LD) 1040 U/L and a total bilirubin of 82 μmol/L, all of which indicated moderate to severe liver damage. I also noted that the patient had recently been treated with atenolol 50 mg daily and that his frusemide dose had doubled to 120 mg twice daily.

I suspected a diagnosis of ischaemic hepatitis, particularly as his AST/LD ratio was 0.93 with clinical evidence of poor peripheral perfusion. So instead of a broadside of antibiotic therapy, I inserted a right heart (Swan Ganz) catheter and took a blood sample for C-reactive protein (CRP).

The cardiac catheter revealed a right atrial pressure of 25 mmHg, pulmonary artery pressure of 70/35 mmHg, pulmonary artery occlusion pressure (PaOP) 31 mmHg and cardiac index of 0.76 L/m^2/min. The CRP level was < 1 mg/L, effectively ruling out 'septic' hepatitis as a diagnosis and indicating a failing heart. A transthoracic echocardiograph was then performed which demonstrated a markedly dilated left ventricle with global dysfunction, a dilated left atrium and right ventricle, moderate mitral regurgitation and mild tricuspid regurgitation.

I phoned the cardiologist and asked "is there any reason why the patient has not been treated with digoxin?"

"The patient's in renal failure, and we rarely, if ever, use digoxin for cardiac failure now," he replied. I thought this a curious comment as atenolol may also be contraindicated in patients with renal failure.

"Have you found the cause of the sepsis?" he added.

"I don't think that the patient is septic" I said. "The CRP is less than 1, the patient is apyrexial, and the biochemistry points more to an ischaemic hepatitis."

"The patient is end-stage then" he said. "Well . . . may not be," I replied. "I'll fiddle with his medications and see how he responds."

"Good luck!" he said. "If you need me I will be on the end of my phone," and with that he hung up.

I decided to treat the patient with captopril syrup 2 mg 4-hourly, increasing over the next few days up to a maximum of 50 mg 8-hourly – if possible – and digoxin 0.75 mg intravenously followed by 0.25 mg after 2 hours and 0.25 mg after 12 hours, to a total dose of 1.25 mg. I also gave the patient one litre of 5% dextrose and 1 litre of 0.9% saline intravenously in the first 24 hours, carefully monitoring the cardiovascular parameters measured by the right heart catheter.

Over the next three days the blood pressure fell from 140/75 to 110/50 mmHg, the PaOP decreased from 31 mmHg to 18 mmHg, the cardiac index increased from 0.76 $L/m^2/min$ to 2.35 $L/m^2/min$ and the right atrial pressure decreased from 25 mmHg to 9 mmHg. A progressive reduction in the plasma ALT, LD and creatinine levels also occurred, indicating an improvement in the perfusion of the liver and kidneys. The blood levels of these compounds returned to normal limits 8 days after his admission.

I reasoned that the patient had had a sudden worsening of his cardiac failure causing the ischaemic hepatitis and renal failure. The deterioration in his heart failure was probably provoked by fluid loss due to vomiting and increased diuretic (frusemide) dose, and was made worse by the atenolol administration, which would have been exacerbated by the progressive renal failure.

When the cardiologist saw the patient again he was amazed at the patient's improvement. He said that digoxin had 'fallen off his radar' in the management of cardiac failure, largely because no drug company promoted it, unlike the newer beta-blockers and renin-angiotensin inhibitors. He added that it was largely the older clinicians who used it, who were possibly not 'up to speed' with the latest treatment of cardiac failure patients. I explained that along with the use of digoxin and careful fluid administration, we were able to increase the dose of captopril and improve the cardiac output. Moreover, I stated that in the management of an acute episode of heart failure, atenolol may have been harmful, particularly in the presence of renal failure.

While he listened courteously, and probably believed that digoxin may have helped, I don't think he was convinced about the adverse effect of the atenolol.

Everything old is new again

"Doctors should file a class action lawsuits against the medical schools because of the flawed education they had received."
Lawrence Weed

"Here's another beauty!" John bellowed.
"Just add water to the canister containing calcium carbide, strike a match to the port at the top and an incandescent light is formed from the acetylene flame. Often used as a light in the early 1900's, but now we use a torch with batteries at three times the cost. I guess that's progress."
We were visiting the outback town of Birdsville, Australia, where John held his audience captive throughout the tour of his unique working museum. Picking through the numerous items used in the early days by those who lived in the bush, he demonstrated to all how to make butter, heal wounds, trap flies, make candles and relieve headaches. All items were innovative, practical and cheap and all able to be made from components that appeared to be readily available from the outback.

One day later I was back at work. It was as though I had not been on a holiday. An eternal number of letters, e-mails and faxes welcomed me. I was also rostered on at the deep end of our group's clinical schedule. Moreover, within the first five minutes I was asked to see an 88 year old lady who 'needed to come to intensive care'.
The patient had been admitted to the A&E department, sweating, cyanosed and struggling for breath. The diagnosis of pulmonary oedema seemed to be likely from her past history of ischaemic heart disease and a history of sudden onset of breathlessness at 4 a.m. that morning. The local medical officer who saw her recorded a pulse rate of 140 beats per minute, blood pressure of 200/120 mmHg and crepitations in all areas of her chest.

L. I. G. Worthley

As I entered the A&E department, the resident doctor rushed to show me a chest X-ray with apical venous congestion and interstitial and alveolar opacities. He also handed me an electrocardiograph which demonstrated sinus rhythm with a left bundle branch block pattern, and an arterial blood gas showing a PaO_2 of 64 mmHg (normally 80 – 100 mmHg), $PaCO_2$ of 58 mmHg (normally 35 – 45 mmHg) and pH of 7.24 (normally 7.35 – 7.45).

"We have started a GTN infusion, given her 80 mg of frusemide and 100% oxygen, but she hasn't improved and I think she needs to come to you," the young doctor eagerly informed me. I probably smiled a little as I vaguely remembered the 'Gomer' in Samuel Shem's 'House of God'.[1]

As I entered the bay to look at the patient, I glanced at the admission sheet and noted that she had not been given any intravenous morphine.

"You didn't give any morphine?" I inquired, and glanced up at the silence to see that I was alone with the patient.

I turned to the lady who was still struggling for breath.

"Mrs. Jones, my name is Dr. Worthley and I've been asked to see you regarding your breathing. In a minute or so, I will give you something that will make you feel a lot better," I said attempting to put her at ease. She closed her eyes and just kept on gasping.

Suddenly, a nurse appeared. Before he could go, I said,

"I wonder if you would draw up 10 mg of morphine and ask the resident to come back please?"

After a few minutes, during which I examined Mrs. Jones to confirm the clinical findings, I was handed a syringe containing the required opiate. The resident doctor returned a minute or two later.

"What do you want me for?" he asked.

"The patient has not been given any morphine so I thought that you may like to see its effect in acute pulmonary oedema," I replied, and without waiting for his response gave the patient the 10 mg as an intravenous bolus.

I looked up at the patient and said, "In a little while your breathing will ease."

The resident blinked in amazement. "Never seen that done before," he mumbled.

"That's a pity," I said. "It's still recommended in the standard texts but nobody seems to use it anymore. I will be back in 10 minutes to see its effect."

I began to walk away with the resident hurrying behind me.

"What happens if she stops breathing?" he said nervously.

"She won't," I replied, and kept on walking.

"But if she does..." he implored.

I stopped, and while feigning composure said quietly "I tell you what, we'll admit her to the ICU if you guarantee that you will come and see her in 30 minutes." I then turned and left.

Thirty minutes later, the resident entered the intensive care unit to see the patient sitting comfortably in bed breathing oxygen at 4 L per minute through nasal cannulae with a pulse oximetry recording of 96%. She was conversing easily and had not required continuous positive airway pressure or endotracheal intubation.

"I guess it's OK for you to use morphine because if they stop breathing then you can intubate them," the young doctor retorted.

"I've not intubated anyone yet with acute pulmonary oedema who is conscious and hypertensive and to whom I've given intravenous morphine," adding "and I use it regularly. You can see the effect it's had in this lady."

The resident shrugged his shoulders and left, although I had a suspicion that this experience had left him none the wiser.

I began wondering about the fate of many of the 'older remedies'. Will morphine for acute pulmonary oedema be relegated to books about ancient medical therapies, in much the same way that digoxin for atrial fibrillation and penicillin for streptococcal infections seem to have been?

Suddenly, I thought of John at the Birdsville working museum.

REFERENCES
1.   Shem S. The House of God. New York: Random House 1979.

At the coalface

"What is freedom of expression? Without the freedom to offend, it ceases to exist."
Salman Rushdie

To graduate as a nurse at the Royal Adelaide Hospital during the 1980's, a period of training in the management of intensive care patients was required during the undergraduate years. These nurses were inexperienced and during their term in the intensive care unit they often appeared like frightened rabbits caught in a spotlight. They did their job dutifully but rarely spoke to the doctor, when he or she entered the ICU bay, and were always under close supervision by the nurse team leader.

I arrived at our intensive care unit early one morning and went to the first bay to find an elderly lady on a ventilator with one of the junior trainee nurses standing by her side. The patient appeared to be intermittently grimacing and extending her arms and legs. Iain, the nurse team leader, quietly entered the room behind me carrying an examination tray.

"Good morning," I said to the trainee nurse and asked "who do we have here?"

"This is Mrs. Jones, doctor. She was admitted last night after visiting her son for dinner, which she often does on Thursday nights. She had not been feeling all that well for most of the day and while she was able to do most of her shopping and house cleaning early in the morning - she even went to her sisters place, which was a little unusual, because her son said that . . . . "

I began to move to the patient's bedside, thinking that the young nurse was presenting a lot of 'chaff' and not much 'wheat'. I slowly picked up the patient's hand. "Go on," I said, not looking at the nurse but concerned more with the intermittent twitching of the patient's hand.

Inside God's Shed

"Well . . . . " she said, and then there was silence. The trainee nurse had probably guessed that I was not particularly interested in her story.

I picked up a pencil on the examination tray and pressed it hard on the patient's nail bed – a standard stimulus often used to assess an unconscious patient's response to pain – and noticed from the corner of my eye the young nurse wincing. I don't know why, perhaps it was just to break the silence, but I thought I would offer a comment.

"I know what you are thinking, you're thinking that he wouldn't do that if it was his mother." She quickly responded. "No, I wasn't thinking that – you see, people like you don't have mothers!"

"Boom boom!" I blurted, and turned to the nurse team leader who couldn't contain his mirth, and was almost in tears while trying to control his laughter. "Iain, what are you teaching these poor students, you've presumably told them that they don't have to stand when we enter the room and don't have to make us tea and scones at the end of the ward round."

Iain knew that I was just trying to provoke the young lass and turned to her and chuckled.

"Don't mind him."

I silently reviewed the case notes and examined the patient for the next 10 minutes, looked at the CT of the brain taken on admission, reviewed her current treatment, increased the sedation and then turned to the nurse and said,

"You're doing a good job."

I then turned and, with Iain, left the room, leaving the junior nurse to tidy the patient's bed.

"A good nurse, Iain? How is she coping?"

"She's OK, I think", he said.

"The patient's had a pretty severe stroke. Did you see the CT?" I asked.

"Yes" he replied. I stopped as we were about to enter the next bay.

"The lady is decerebate, and will probably last no more than a day or so before she becomes brain dead. Will the trainee nurse be good with that?" I asked.

"I think so." Iain then thought for a moment and added,

"perhaps I'll put her with one of the post-op vascular patients; they always make a good recovery. She'll like that more."

During my time as an intensivist I found the ICU nursing staff were second to none. They were hard-working, professional and genuinely loved their patients. Their training was long and arduous, although some, understandably, did not enjoy the high mortality rate often found in our units. Care of the dying is difficult and requires a special skill. For those without the temperament to manage these patients, there will be other specialties that are equally rewarding (e.g. obstetrics and pediatrics) where death and dying are rare.

The checklist is not something new

"ICU's that are run by protocols can be run by monkeys – and usually are."
L. I. G. Worthley[1]

"With our large patient load we have a window of opportunity to design and study protocols that deliver best practice to the ICU patient. Protocols for diagnosis – you know, investigating pyrexia, and tachycardia, and hypoxia and a whole lot of other things, as well as protocols and checklists for treatment, like a standard approach for ventilating a patient, or fluid and electrolyte management – all evidence-based stuff. What about it, Tub?"

"Sounds good, Bob" I said, trying to sound enthusiastic.

It was another whirlwind bright idea from a newly appointed head of the department of anaesthesia and intensive care, using the same jargon of 'evidence-based' and 'best practice' interspersed with the usual clichés of 'window of opportunity' that we hear each month when he attends our ward round. Initially, we acted upon these 'bright ideas'. One of which was "lets change our ICU monitoring system to current best practice – we have a window of opportunity as the money's available if we use it before the end of the financial year." We wasted hours reviewing equipment and writing up a tender only to have the project shelved. These boondoggles were either the dreams of an unrealistic mind, or schemes to keep the minions busy and away from any subversive activity.

Nevertheless, as far as the head of the department was concerned, checklists, protocols and guidelines were here to stay, so we better get cracking. I remember visiting one Australasian intensive care unit where the staff were endeavouring to manage patients using a heavy dose of these tools. It seemed to me that the unit didn't need intensivists, the patient could be managed by robots. No training necessary; just program the resident medical officer with protocols – the consultant could be dismissed.

While we discussed the strengths and weaknesses of these routines, I began to realize that some of our procedures were already codified as checklists and had been working well for many years. It was nothing new or revolutionary. For example, we used a checklist for the diagnosis of brain death. A checklist was used for the investigation of atypical pneumonia.[2] Other medical checklists had also been developed, including checklists to reduce deep vein thrombosis and pulmonary embolism, acute gastric erosions, hyperglycaemia, malnutrition and vitamin deficiency. These required subcutaneous injections of heparin twice a day, an intravenous proton pump inhibitor, a sliding insulin scale, enteral or parenteral nutrition and intravenous vitamins. Moreover, as muscle wasting, bone atrophy and limb, mouth and eye ulcers were problems in the unconscious ICU patient, nursing checklists had been designed and used for years to reduce these complications. Joints and muscles were stretched to avoid contractures, patients were turned in bed and limbs repositioned every few hours to reduce pressure sores. Also the body, teeth and mouth were washed and eyelids taped closed, all of which were scheduled regularly 6 – 12 hourly and recorded in the nursing chart when completed.

Anaesthetists use a checklist before beginning an anaesthetic, checking the anaesthetic machine, monitoring devices, oxygen supply, flowmeters, vaporizers, breathing system, inspiratory and expiratory valves, mechanical ventilator, bag-and-mask, etc, etc, to ensure all are ready and functioning properly before anaesthetizing the patient.[3] The ICU nurse performs a similar checklist when preparing an ICU bay ready for a patient. Before operating, the surgeon checks that the correct patient is about to be anaesthetized, the operation to be performed is correct and that the consent form has been signed.[4]

Humans have used checklists as memory aids for centuries. Physicians have employed mnemonics to remember countless nerve and arterial branches for the last 80 years[5] using a publication that can now be downloaded free from the internet.[6] I remember 40 years ago filling a number of little black books with lists of clinical features, diagnostic tests and treatments for a myriad of rare diseases to use as an aide-mémoire in answering postgraduate examination questions.

Inside God's Shed

However, checklists are not a panacea. They are developed as a memory aid when tedious and uninspiring procedures lead to a thoughtless omission of an important step. When found to be of benefit they become established,[7] although they do not always correlate directly with a reduction in human error and improvement in patient care.[8] Fundamentally, they are not a solution to substandard medical training.

A large prospective study reported a sustained reduction of up to 60% in rates of central venous catheter (CVC) related bloodstream infections by implementing a checklist of: 1) appropriate hand hygiene, 2) use of 2% chlorhexidine for skin preparation, 3) use of full-barrier precautions during the catheter insertion, 4) subclavian vein placement as the preferred site, and 5) removing unnecessary central venous catheters.[9] However, the study was not randomised or controlled, antibiotic or antiseptic coated catheters – which are now used routinely – were not used, and it is not clear how many hospitals enrolled in the study had staff who previously used an appropriate standard of care when inserting a CVC. These five steps, along with other important tasks, should be routine for CVC insertions without using a checklist.[10] One could conclude that instead of a checklist, practitioners undertaking CVC insertions at these institutions should be retrained.

There are other important limitations with protocols and checklists that have been previously described.[11,12] However, and importantly, rather than having a filing cabinet full of protocols, checklists and guidelines, each institution should have an active intensive care medicine education and research program, as they provide the environment necessary to enforce a safe and appropriate acute care practice.

What happened to the protocols, checklists and guidelines that were developed at our intensive care unit? I believe that the majority of paperwork we generated gathers dust at the bottom of a drawer somewhere. One of the major 'window of opportunity' checklists that were developed was a withdrawal-of-therapy protocol that required signatures of the next of kin or medical power of attorney, admitting consultant, intensivist, and administrator – or representative. It was subsequently used in a case that went to court and found to be most unhelpful. It, along with the other tools, are now no longer used.

REFERENCES
1. Worthley LIG. The power of the clinical examination - back to the future. 19th Australian and New Zealand Scientific Meeting on Intensive Care. Sydney, October 1994.
2. Worthley LIG. Synopsis of Intensive Care Medicine. London: Churchill Livingstone, 1994; p942.
3. The Association of Anaesthetists of Great Britain and Ireland – Checklist for anaesthetic equipment 2004. www.aagbi.org/sites/default/files/checklista404.pdf. (accessed April 2012).
4. WHO Surgical safety checklist (first edition). http://www.who.int/patientsafety/safesurgery/ss_checklist/en/. (accessed April 2012).
5. Irving AS. Anatomy mnemonics. Churchill Livingstone: Edinburgh 1939.
6. Smith AG. Anatomy mnemonics. Irving's anatomy mnemonics. www.similima.com/books/irving-anatomy-mnemonics.pdf. (accessed April 2012).
7. Hales B, Terblanche M, Fowler R, Sibbald W. Development of medical checklists for improved quality of patient care. Int J Qual Health Care 2008;20:22-30.
8. Manley R, Cuddeford JD. An assessment of the effectiveness of the revised FDA checklist. AANA J 1966;64:277-282.
9. Pronovost P, Needham D, Berenholtz S,. Sinopoli D, Chu H, Cosgrove S, et al. An intervention to decrease catheter-related bloodstream infections in the ICU. N Engl J Med 2006;355:2725-2732.
10. Braner DAV, Lai S, Eman S, Tegtmeyer K. Central venous catheterization - subclavian vein. N Engl J Med 2007; 357:e26.
11. Leape LL. Error in medicine. JAMA 1994;272:1851-1857.
12. Ingelfinger FJ. Algorithms, anyone? N Engl J Med 1973;288:847-848.

"Could we have a second opinion?"

"My psychiatrist told me I was crazy and I said I want a second opinion. He said okay, you're ugly too."
Rodney Danderfield

The request for a second opinion by the relatives of an unconscious patient in the intensive care unit is rare, and I was somewhat surprised, when recently I outlined to a mother the diagnosis, plan and prognosis for her severely head injured son, to be asked 'could we have a second opinion?'

The patient had just been admitted to the ICU after a motor vehicle accident in which his only major lesion was a closed head injury. He arrived at the hospital A&E department deeply unconscious with a Glasgow Coma Score of 7. He was intubated and mechanically ventilated and underwent a cerebral CT scan which revealed bifrontal lobe contusions and early signs of cerebral oedema. The on-call neurosurgical team assessed the patient, inserted an intracranial pressure (ICP) monitor and referred him to the ICU team for further management. I told the mother that her son had a severe head injury with signs of brain damage and that there was evidence of increased pressure inside his head, which was not a particularly good sign, although it was early in the course of his illness and that the final outcome could not be predicted with any certainty. On one hand, he could make a very good recovery, yet on the other hand he could be severely disabled; we just had to wait and review his progress daily.

"Was there anything more that could be done?" "Is there any centre in the world that specialises in head injuries where we could send him?" "Please spare no expense," were just a few of the many questions and comments that were rattled off by a genuinely concerned divorced mother who had reared her son without any help from a father who had long gone.

I explained to her that at our institution we had a lot of experience in dealing with head-injured patients and, as a teaching hospital, we constantly reviewed world literature to keep in touch with recent developments. We knew what was available and genuinely believed that the patient would not benefit from being moved to another centre. The ICU team consisted of 5 specialists, all of whom would be either directly or indirectly involved in her son's care, and all of whom would ensure that an excellence in care would be maintained.

Later that day she returned with her sister and two brothers, and asked me to go through what I had said to her - to all of them. This I did, attempting to make sure that the dialogue was honest, unhurried and almost identical with that which I had relayed some four hours earlier. At the end I looked at them and asked "are there any questions?" The mother looked at me and said "please don't misunderstand us, as we know that Kevin is receiving the best care possible, but could we have a second opinion?"

"Sure" I said, not wanting to appear obstructive. "As I said, we solicit opinions from all our ICU specialists when dealing with critically ill patients – so what had you in mind?" I wanted to reassure her we consulted widely, but did not want her to feel she was losing control of her right to another opinion.

It appeared that her sister knew a neurosurgeon at another hospital and wondered whether he could provide the second opinion.

"Sure" I said again. "I know him well, and will give him a call. We would be happy for him to be involved." I quickly informed our neurosurgical team of these developments, and a cryptic message was relayed back: "do what you like. The current management is non-surgical."

The second opinion arrived two days later and deep into the evening. The patient by this time was heavily sedated with morphine and midazolam. He was non-responsive to pain, had pinpoint pupils and a cerebral CT scan performed that morning revealed a generalised increase in cerebral oedema but no surgically remedial lesion. His ICP had been varying between 17 - 20 mmHg, the serum osmolality was 305 mOsm/kg (increasing over the last 24 hr due to intermittent osmotherapy) and the arterial PaO_2 and $PaCO_2$ were 116 mmHg and 36 mmHg, respectively. The consultation was brief. Unfortunately, no 'on site' medical staff knew of his presence, so he remained unaccompanied throughout. Next morning the 'advice' was noticed in the case record, which included hyperventilating the patient down to a $PaCO_2$ of 25 - 30 mmHg, intravenous dexamethasone 8 mg 4-hourly and thiopentone until the ICP was below 15 mmHg, while administering noradrenaline and intravenous fluids if the cerebral perfusion pressure fell below 70 mmHg. These recommendations had also been relayed by the neurosurgeon to the mother via her sister, so that by early morning we were confronted with an enthusiastic family believing that a formula had been found which would somehow transform their boy rapidly into an awake and vibrant individual. I remembered telling the family the previous day that everything that could be done was being done. How could this be reconciled with steroids, thiopentone and hyperventilation?

To say that I was a little irritated at the second opinion's advice and method of communication was putting it mildly. "We were thankful for these added thoughts," I said suppressing my ire, "and were aware of these treatments. However, we had not used them because large trials involving many patients with an injury similar to your son's, have shown them to be of little use."

"But what have we got to lose?" was the cry from a mother desperate to try anything.

"Well . . . side-effects can occur, which are not insignificant, and may cause more harm than good," I said in an attempt to justify what was appearing to be a therapeutically nihilistic position.

"What about trying it?" was all she could say.

"What we will do," I said, attempting to reach middle ground, "will be to introduce each of these suggested therapies carefully, but will withdraw them if there seems to be any adverse effects." She seemed relieved.

"Unless you would prefer us to send Kevin to a hospital where the other neurosurgeon could continue his management," I said hastily, wanting to allow her all options concerning her son's treatment, and allowing the 'second opinion' to deal with the problem at first hand.

"Oh no! We are perfectly happy with your management. We would just like to make sure that no stone is left unturned" – a puzzling statement that I thought best left unchallenged.

L. I. G. Worthley

As it would happen (perhaps fortuitously) my rostered 'week on' for the ward was almost over, and I handed over to a consultant who was less troubled than I about the external control of management of this head-injured boy. I introduced him to the family, saying that I had acquainted him with all the relevant facts and that further management would be under his 'watchful eye'.

However, I could not forget this episode. I kept wondering about the second opinion and its value in medicine. When doctors consult, the advice is usually received gratefully, with the referring doctor taking up some or all of the suggested changes in the patient's management. The relatives are informed of the suggested changes with the referring doctor discussing the advantages and disadvantages of each; rarely are they directly involved in the consultation process. Consultation differs from a 'second opinion' in that the latter is usually initiated by a patient or relative who is unhappy with the first opinion, which not only relates to the advice given, but also to the relationship developed between patient or relative and doctor.[1,2] Concerning the advice, both the reliability and reproducibility of clinical judgement vary with time, indicating that the doctor giving the 'second opinion' varies his or her advice with time.[3] Concerning the doctor-patient relationship, this is a matter of trust, which is an essential, but fragile, element of good medical care,[4] and while it commonly does not vary over time, when a second opinion is requested it can easily deteriorate.

If the patient wishes to undergo treatment recommended by the second doctor, clearly the management should be taken over by that doctor. It would seem that continued management by the first doctor undertaking management advised by the second doctor would be unworkable. Who then is responsible for the patient's management? Who is liable for adverse effects or treatment failures?

While a second opinion is a patient's 'right', as a tool it has to be used carefully.

REFERENCES
1. Sutherland LR, Verhoef MJ. Why do patients seek a second opinion or alternative medicine? J Clin Gastroenterol 1994;19:194-197.

2. Sutherland LR, Verhoef MJ. Patients who seek a second opinion: are they different from the typical referral? J Clin Gastroenterol 1989;11:308-313.
3. Rutkow IM. Surgical decision making. The reproducibility of clinical judgement. Arch Surg 1982;117:337-340.
4. Relman AS. Practicing medicine in the new business climate. N Engl J Med 1987;316:1150-1151.

Peanuts, pain, purgatory and persistence – at a price

"Nothing in this world can take the place of persistence. Talent will not; nothing is more common than unsuccessful men with talent. Genius will not, unrewarded genius is almost a proverb. Education will not, the world is full of educated derelicts. Persistence and determination alone are omnipotent."
   Calvin Coolidge

I first met the Australian cricketer Neil Hawke many years ago at the start of a long and erratic medical saga. To be exact, it was 8 p.m. on the 9th July 1980. I was holding one side of a Jordan frame lifter preparing to slide him from the ambulance stretcher onto the intensive care unit admission bay bed. He was cyanosed, shivering and grimaced with pain every time he moved. This was 24 hours after a laparotomy had been performed at Modbury Hospital for an acute bowel obstruction.

Neil had a past medical history of a difficult retrocaecal appendicectomy in 1960, and an intestinal obstruction after eating peanuts in 1976. The latter was treated surgically at the Burnley General Hospital in the UK, with a right paramedian laparotomy and division of multiple adhesions. Seven days later an incisional hernia developed which was finally repaired in 1978 with the insertion of a Marlex® mesh patch.

The current bowel obstruction was also caused by eating peanuts, which Neil consumed continuously on Saturday 5th July as he watched the 1980 Wimbledon tennis final between John McEnroe and Björn Borg. Within twelve hours he developed severe abdominal pain and was admitted to Modbury Hospital where he was treated with nasogastric suction, nil by mouth and intravenous fluids.

While he initially improved his abdominal pain persisted, so a laparotomy was deemed necessary for further management.

Inside God's Shed

On 8th July, he underwent a laparotomy via a left paramedian incision – to avoid the right-sided Marlex® mesh patch – with division of multiple adhesions, and oversewing of an inadvertent defect in the small bowel that occurred when sharp dissection was used to free the densely adherent bowel from the back of the previous operation scar. An inspissated peanut mass causing the small bowel obstruction was found proximal to one of the adhesions. The adhesion was divided and the peanut mass was allowed to pass through.

Six hours later Neil had increasing abdominal pain with intermittent rigors. He had not passed urine for the previous 4 hours and became progressively more breathless and disorientated. His temperature was 40°C, blood pressure 70/30 mmHg and pulse rate 145 beats per minute, so he was transferred to the intensive care unit at the Royal Adelaide Hospital for dialysis and ongoing management.

Fred (the ICU director) was at the head of the lifter and ordered "Shift on the count of three. One – two – three – shift!" and, with a muffled cry from Neil, he was moved from the stretcher to the bed. We wheeled him to an isolation bay, inserted a right heart catheter, arterial line, placed cardiac leads on his chest and reviewed his vital signs and recent blood results. The blood cultures taken at Modbury Hospital from the previous day revealed a positive culture of mixed organisms including *Bacteroides* spp, *Clostridium perfringens* and *E. coli*. The plasma biochemistry showed elevated levels of bilirubin, creatinine, urea, potassium, phosphate and liver enzymes, and low levels of calcium and sodium. He was anaemic with low white cell and platelet counts and his arterial blood gases revealed a metabolic acidosis with low oxygen and carbon dioxide levels. In brief he had severe, if not lethal, multiple organ failure with a mixed organism septicaemia and circulatory shock.

While the surgical team believed that he was not fit for surgery, we convinced them that he would die if nothing more were done. His only chance of surviving, we argued, would be the correction of any surgically remediable abdominal lesion.

Two hours later, and following a brief period of resuscitation with fluids, inotropic agents and antibiotics, a laparotomy was performed. This exposed a perforation at the previously oversewn small bowel site, two segments of gangrenous small bowel, and large necrotic areas of subcutaneous fat and rectus muscle. The gangrenous small bowel was removed and the necrotic subcutaneous fat and rectus muscle were excised. Subsequent histology of the rectus muscle revealed gas gangrene. As the abdominal muscle and subcutaneous fat were unable to be opposed, skin juxtaposition only, using mattress sutures, provided closure of the abdominal cavity. Postoperatively, he was returned to the ICU, mechanically ventilated, on 100% oxygen and on high doses of inotropic agents. His dry skin was a grey-yellow colour; he had poor peripheral perfusion and was deeply unconscious. An arterio-venous shunt was inserted and dialysis commenced.

On the 12th July, the skin sutures were removed, the wound gaped and a large portion of small intestine was exposed. The exposed bowel was covered with saline packs that were changed daily for the next six days. On the 18th July, the abdominal defect was re-sutured and a tracheostomy was performed to facilitate tracheal suction and prolonged mechanical ventilation. He remained in a coma for three weeks, needed inotropic support for four weeks, daily dialysis for seven weeks and mechanical ventilation for 5 months.

During the first six months Neil endured many critical episodes. For example on:

21st July – he suffered gastric bleeding from confluent gastric stress ulcers, requiring a 17 unit blood transfusion, 4 units of fresh frozen plasma and 4 packs of platelets.

22nd July – he required a laparotomy and oversewing of two small bowel perforations, following which the abdominal wound was left open revealing peristalting bowel underneath.

26th July – two more small bowel fistulae developed.

14th September – a total of 5 small bowel fistulae and a gastric fistula were drained and dressed daily.

2nd October – in an attempt to epithelialise the gaping abdominal wound, a split skin graft from his left thigh was placed directly onto the exposed small bowel wall.

10th October – a massive gastric haemorrhage occurred requiring transfusion of 28 units of blood, 6 units of fresh frozen plasma and 8 packs of platelets. An operative exploration of the abdomen exposed a

Inside God's Shed

necrotic anterior wall of the stomach and two large bleeding arterial vessels at the base of a large gastric erosion. The bleeding arterial vessels were oversewn and the stomach was packed with saline and adrenaline soaked packs. The packs were replaced three times during the next 12 hours. A total of 40 units of blood were transfused during this episode.

During this period Neil remained severely jaundiced, with a chronic superficial pseudomonas infection on the surface of the exposed bowel, as well as in numerous small ulcers on his back. A chronic sacral bed sore developed and became infected with a mixed growth of methicillin resistant *Staphylococcus aureus* and *Pseudomonas aeruginosa*. He had a penicillin and cephalosporin allergic reaction causing an exfoliative dermatitis. A urethral fistula developed through the scrotum. He had six asystolic cardiac arrests and numerous episodes of sinus bradycardia induced by two doses of intravenous cimetidine. Numerous central venous line infections with *Staphylococcus epidermidis* occurred which were successfully treated by using a small dose of hydrochloric acid (1 mL 2N HCl) directly instilled into the silastic catheter.[1] He also developed carnitine deficiency, which was corrected by adding a dose of carnitine to his nightly intravenous nutrition.[2]

The tracheostomy caused a tracheal stenosis, so on the 12th February 1981 the stenotic segment was removed and the trachea was re-anastomosed with the addition of a chin-to-sternum suture to provide minimal tension on the trachea. The suture was removed after two weeks and over the next four weeks the neck flexion was slowly increased to allow the trachea to gently stretch.

Three feet of small bowel were resected on the 24th April 1981 and an end-to-end anastomosis from the jejunum to the distal small bowel allowed the removal of five small bowel fistulae with one gastric fistula remaining. As the skin grafts had derived their blood supply from the underlying bowel, the abdominal skin sloughed, requiring another split skin graft from the left thigh to re-epithelialize the exposed bowel wall. His convalescence following this operation was prolonged, as his mobilisation was impaired due to the development of critical illness polyneuropathy and postural hypotension. The latter required an abdominal binder to reduce the venous pooling within the abdomen when he stood. His lower limb muscle strength slowly returned using a mobile quadrapod and a comprehensive series of exercises.

After an eleven month period in the intensive care unit he was discharged home for three months to improve his physical and mental condition. The gastric fistula was cared for by his wife, Bev, and the home parenteral nutrition was managed with weekly blood analysis and home visits. Finally, the gastric fistula was closed surgically and a pseudomonas-infected xiphisternum was removed. While he had a short period of postoperative sepsis, he slowly improved to ultimately have his central venous line removed and oral nutrition introduced.

During this time I discovered his sense of humour. When he was ill I was often required to perform a procedure that would inevitably cause pain. He may have grimaced, but he never uttered a harsh word. One year later, after he had been discharged from hospital and was again enjoying life, I was admitted to hospital for an ear operation. He and Bev were my first visitors. I remember the cheeky look he gave me as he poked his head around the doorway of my hospital room. "G'day mate," he grinned, then bellowed, "Nurse get me a syringe! One with a big blunt needle!" His face beamed as he chuckled.

His acute illness had extended from the 9th July 1980 until the 10th August 1982, during which time he received a total of 232 units of blood (approximately 110 litres), 45 units of fresh frozen plasma (approximately 12 litres), 72 packs of platelets and a large amount of human albumin. He was left with cirrhosis of the liver, a staghorn kidney calculus, hepatitis B and C infections and chronic cerebellar degeneration that limited his speech and mobility.

In 1991, I moved to the Flinders Medical Centre and thereafter had only intermittent contact with Neil. His care now required other specialists as he developed hepatic failure (from transfusion-induced hepatitis B and C infections), chronic renal failure and a disabling encephalopathy. More treatment was required, but over the remaining years it became clear that his time was slowly drawing to a close.

I saw him on three occasions at the Mary Potter Hospice. Death, now a kindly old friend, was not far away. While Neil's words were more measured and his movements slower, he still had a twinkle in his eye. His body had clearly aged and had started to give way to the ravages of disease. Nevertheless, his spirit remained young as ever. It was good to talk, once again, to a very dear friend.

Neil James Napier Hawke was born 27th June 1939 and died 25th December 2000; he lived for almost 20 years following his abdominal catastrophe. I was asked to speak at his memorial service which was held at the Assemblies of God Church at Paradise, Adelaide, on Friday 29th December 2000, saying:

"It is unusual that in such a crippling illness, one finds a mind and body so dominated by a desire to overcome a never-ending series of normally lethal conditions, to persist against such overwhelming odds and to slowly but surely climb over each barrier to finally become independent and well. Even during the bleakest of times, both he and Bev believed that he would endure. She would tend his stomach wounds, which leaked putrid fluids that would often need to be dealt with at the most inopportune times, forever unhurried, always with a gentle touch and with tender devotion. I won't proceed to detail that dreadful year of torment that both he and Bev suffered; suffice to say that it finally ended. He, with an unbelievable inner strength fired by a genuine love of life, had beaten the odds.

I have often been given the credit for Neil's survival, when clearly it has been others who deserve whatever credit is given. Medically, there has been a cast of thousands, some of whom Neil had outlived. More importantly, however, it was the combination of the mental, physical and spiritual fortitude that Neil innately possessed, combined with Bev's unswerving care. To him she was an angel that always appeared from a sea of despair, both were necessary for him to be given those extra 20 years of life.

To every thing there is a season, and a time to every purpose under the heaven. Goodbye Neil, we will be with you again soon. You are now at peace."

Throughout his illness, a few doctors at the periphery of his management believed that "he should be allowed to die". When we asked "why?" we would be told, "because it is not in his best interests"; an answer that held little meaning to a determined patient

L. I. G. Worthley

and a loving wife. All clinicians are well aware that in a prolonged life-threatening illness, death can be the final outcome, but there is also no doubt that if a team of unwilling professionals are involved it will be a certainty.

REFERENCES
1. Worthley LIG. Treatment of central venous silastic catheter infections using hydrochloric acid. Anaesth Intensive Care 1982;10:314-318.
2. Worthley LIG, Fishlock RC, Snoswell AM. Carnitine deficiency with hyperbilirubinaemia, generalized skeletal muscle weakness and reactive hypoglycaemia in a patient on long term total parenteral nutrition: Treatment with intravenous L-carnitine. J Parenter Enteral Nutr 1983;7:176-180.

If you tread on another intensivist's shoes – do it softly

"I often regret that I have spoken; never that I have been silent."
Publilius Syrus

"Tub, what do you think about giving glucose and insulin for a diltiazem overdose?" asked our senior registrar.

"Sounds good, mate" I replied. It was not my rostered week 'on' in the public hospital ICU, and the last thing an off duty intensivist should do is to stick his nose in another intensivist's area of responsibility. So I gave a word or two of encouragement without offering any uninvited advice. The registrar persisted,

"We are having some trouble with a lady who was admitted to the ICU a day ago after taking a total of 5.76 grams of slow release diltiazem capsules. She's still bradycardic and hypotensive despite large doses of adrenaline and noradrenaline."

The registrar waited for my response. Finally I said,

"What does David (the on duty intensivist) think about this?" as I was still a little reticent about cutting across his line of responsibility.

"Well, he's just put her on vasopressin to get the blood pressure up – which has made absolutely no difference," said the registrar now sounding a little frustrated.

"Where's the patient?" I asked reluctantly.

"She's just around the corner."

We both went to her bedside. On examination she was drowsy but orientated. Her blood pressure was 80/50 mmHg and pulse rate was 40 beats per minute. I noted that she had been given calcium chloride, glucagon and 0.9% saline on admission, which increased her blood pressure slightly but her pulse remained at 40 beats per minute, which persisted in spite of the addition of adrenaline, noradrenaline and now vasopressin.

During any calcium channel blocker (e.g. diltiazem, verapamil, nifedipine or amlodipine) overdose, pancreatic beta cell insulin secretion is inhibited,[1] causing hypoinsulinaemia and a reduction in cellular entry of glucose. Glucose and insulin infusions have been used to treat experimental cardiac depression associated with verapamil poisoning,[1] and in clinical reports of severe diltiazem, verapamil and amlodipine poisoning, a continuous infusion of insulin up to 35 U/hr and glucose have been used successfully to manage these patients.[2,3,4,5]

"I reckon that an infusion of insulin and dextrose is worth a go," I said, "but I wouldn't ask David first because he might say 'no' and then you would be 'buggered'. As you are the senior registrar on duty, I would just do it and tell him later. David won't mind you doing it, but he'd be troubled if he knew I was involved – so don't tell him."

I then asked, "What are you planning to do?" as I felt some responsibility in overseeing the treatment, even if obliquely, just in case the registrar was about to embark upon a thoroughly hair-brained plan of management.

"Well" he said, "I think I will infuse Actrapid® at 5 U/hr increasing to 25 U/hr over 1 to 2 hours and infuse 50% dextrose to keep the plasma glucose levels varying between 6 - 8 mmol/L. I'll do a blood sugar level every ½ hour for the first few hours and when the levels are stable, probably reduce that to hourly."

"Sounds good," I said.

Within 30 minutes of the insulin infusion reaching 25 U/hr, the blood pressure had increased to 120/60 mmHg. After a further 30 minutes, the adrenaline, noradrenaline and vasopressin infusions were discontinued. The insulin infusion was continued at 25 U/hr for a further 6 hours then reduced to 10 U/hr for 2 hours. Thereafter the 50% dextrose was discontinued and the insulin varied between 0 - 4 U/hr to keep the plasma glucose level varying between 6 - 8 mmol/L.

Both the senior registrar and the on call intensivist reported the successful outcome of this therapy at the evening ward round. I got a smile from the senior registrar during the presentation. Everybody was happy.

REFERENCES
1. Kline JA, Leonova E, Raymond RM. Beneficial myocardial metabolic effects of insulin during verapamil toxicity in the anesthetized canine. Crit Care Med 1995;23:1251-1263.
2. Yuan TH, Herns WP, Tomaszewski CA, Ford MD, Kline JA. Insulin-glucose as adjunctive therapy for severe calcium channel antagonist poisoning. J Toxicol Clin Toxicol 1999;37:463-474.
3. Boyer EW, Shannon M. Treatment of calcium-channel-blocker intoxication with insulin infusion. N Engl J Med 2001;344:1721-1722.
4. Rasmussen L, Husted SE, Johnsen SP. Severe intoxication after an intentional overdose of amlodipine. Acta Anaesthesiol Scand 2003;47:1038-1040.
5. Boyer EW, Duic PA, Evans A. Hyperinsulinemia/euglycemia therapy for calcium channel blocker poisoning. Pediatr Emerg Care 2002;18:36-37.

Shhh! I think it's the patient

"The true antithesis of 'caring medicine' is not 'scientific medicine' or 'high technology medicine' or 'hospital medicine' or 'academic medicine' or 'orthodox medicine' it is quite simply 'bad medicine.'"
Douglas A. K. Black

As the indication for an admission to an intensive care unit is the development of a 'sudden or potentially sudden and reversible life-threatening condition', not all patients are unconscious and on 'life support' (i.e. intubated and mechanically ventilated), they may even be fully conscious and spontaneously breathing. Nevertheless, many require some form of respiratory assistance, and the patient's conscious state usually varies from being drowsy to deeply unconscious.

The variation in consciousness can be caused by sedative, opiate or tranquilising drugs producing an 'induced coma', or caused by disease from stroke, cerebral trauma, encephalitis, meningitis, etc. Rarely the patient may be alert but paralysed, and appear to be 'asleep' but is frighteningly conscious and unable to move. This is the 'nightmare' event that sporadically occurs during operative surgery when a relaxant anaesthetic provides paralysis in the absence of adequate analgesia and sedation. This is known as intra-operative awareness, although in the intensive care patient it can be caused by neurological diseases, where the patient has lost all muscle power but remains conscious and alert; a condition known as 'locked-in syndrome'.[1]

Intensive care specialists share many of the skills anaesthetists have when they provide anaesthesia and resuscitation to surgical patients in theatre. However, as there is usually no constant surgical stimulus experienced by the ICU patient, the current trend in managing intensive care patients on 'life support' is to provide less anaesthesia than that necessary for an operation. This is important as total mechanical ventilation using paralysing drugs is now thought to be less desirable for lung function and repair, than partial mechanical support where the patient provides some of the effort in breathing.[2,3] Analgesia and sedation are now tailored to facilitate varying degrees of mechanical ventilation while ensuring the patient is comfortable and, to some extent, alert. Clinical examination of the patient is also less compromised when compared with deep anaesthesia, allowing the clinician to assess the presence of abnormal symptoms and signs.

"But the patient is intubated and not moving so communication is impossible," the junior doctor or nurse may say.

Is this true? While interaction with the patient may be limited, they are often able to feel, hear and even see. When a clinician or nurse examines the patient at the bedside, a reassuring touch or sound from a practitioner will be interpreted as being treated by one who cares – a vital reassurance to the patient who may be wondering, in his or her sedated and disorientated state, what will befall them – in this worrisome place. The emotional condition of a patient is still as important as any single factor in the treatment of disease and is probably more so when technology abounds.

I sometimes wonder if certain clinicians are drawn to the specialty of intensive care medicine because it reduces their exposure to a talking patient. However the intensivist will be required to discuss the critically ill patient's condition in great detail, if not to the patient, to the relatives. This requires a suitably skilled communicator particularly if the patient has a reduced chance of survival.

Brain death, especially in the young, and when unexpected, requires many conversing skills, not only in discussing exactly what is happening and what the future holds,[4] but also in taking the relatives carefully through the minefield of the 'body alive but brain dead' concept;[5] and then raising the topic of organ donation.

REFERENCES
1. Smith E, Delargy M. Locked-in syndrome. BMJ 2005;330:406-409.
2. Worthley LIG, Fisher MMcD. The fat embolism syndrome treated with oxygen, diuretics, sodium restriction, and spontaneous ventilation. Anaesth Intens Care 1979;7:136-142.
3. Antonelli M, Conti G, Rocco M, Bufi M, De Blasi RA, Vivino G, et al. A comparison of noninvasive positive-pressure ventilation

and conventional mechanical ventilation in patients with acute respiratory failure. N Engl J Med 1998;339:429-435.
4. Wijdicks EFM. Current concepts: the diagnosis of brain death. N Engl J Med 2001;344:1215-1221.
5. Shewmon DA. Chronic "brain death"; a meta-analysis and conceptual consequences. Neurology 1998;51:1538-1545.

Please read the fine print

"Learning without thought is labour lost; thought without learning is perilous."
Confucius

I was called to see a patient who had just been admitted to the intensive care unit from one of the general wards, and entered the patient's bay just after he had been intubated and ventilated. The medical registrar was at the end of the bed looking at the patient's electrocardiogram, the ICU registrar was securing the endotracheal tube, and the nursing staff were busy preparing to set up for an arterial line and a Swan Ganz catheter insertion.

The ICU registrar looked up, raised his eyebrows and smiled a little as he began to tell me the story. The patient was an 86 year old man with severe ischaemic heart disease, chronic atrial fibrillation and mitral valve disease who had had numerous episodes of pulmonary oedema over the past 12 years. His medications included perindopril, digoxin, frusemide, amlodipine, spironolactone, warfarin and amiodarone. He had been admitted to a medical ward three days ago with a two day history of increasing shortness of breath and resistant peripheral oedema. However, while he had improved with continuous positive airway pressure, graduating to oxygen at 4 L/min via nasal cannulae, during the morning of the third day he became progressively more short of breath and hypotensive. When the ICU team arrived in response to a 'medical emergency' call, he had marked cyanosis and was gasping.

As the ICU registrar appeared to have the clinical situation under control and as a 'Swan' and an arterial line were about to be inserted, I decided to review the case notes quietly in a corner.

It appeared that during his three-day inpatient workup, the chest X-ray showed a large heart in failure, and the plasma biochemistry revealed a resolving ischaemic hepatitis, with an INR decreasing from 8.2 to 3.3, and an improvement in renal function with the creatinine

57

decreasing from 0.52 mmol/L to 0.46 mmol/L. The echocardiograph confirmed severe global left ventricular dysfunction with mitral regurgitation. I also noticed that one hour before the ICU team was called he was given carvedilol 3.125 mg orally.

"Why was he given carvedilol?" I asked.

"To help his heart failure," replied the medical registrar, as he continued to peruse the ECG. He quickly followed with "the latest 'New England Journal of Medicine' reported a huge multicentre trial where carvedilol reduced the mortality of patients who had grade IV heart failure."

"Nice study, but didn't it exclude patients with renal failure?" I inquired provocatively.

The registrar immediately looked up, probably to assess whether he was talking to a 'true believer' or not.

"Patients with renal failure were included," he blurted, and nervously began to fidget with his stethoscope.

At this stage we both knew that the important features of this study were a little hazy in both our minds, but I can remember thinking, as I read the article, that carvedilol was not an agent that we would be using often in our critically ill population. While I would accept that adrenergic stimulation has a maladaptive role in chronic heart failure, and that trials of beta-blockade – orally and in gradually escalating doses – have reported beneficial effects in clinically stable patients, in critically ill patients who have severe systolic heart failure, beta-adrenergic receptor blockade (e.g. using carvedilol) can be hazardous.

Later that day I wandered back to my office and logged onto www.nejm.org and found the article in question, which appeared in the 31st May 2001 edition.[1] The patient who was admitted to the ICU would have been excluded from that trial for many reasons, including being a hospitalised patient with an acute cardiac illness requiring continuous inpatient care, severe peripheral oedema, renal failure (i.e. serum creatinine > 0.248 mmol/L) and receiving a calcium channel blocker (i.e. amlodipine).

Such broad interpretations of various 'landmark' articles with little consideration given to the exclusion criteria, i.e. failure to read the fine print, are not necessarily rare. Some clinicians do not restore a haemoglobin level beyond 70 g/L in acutely ill patients because in a recent study 'mortality was not improved with transfusion'.[2] However, they ignore the exclusion criteria of: a decrease in haemoglobin of 30 g/L in the preceding 12 hours, requirement of 3 or more units of packed cells in the preceding 12 hours and postoperative cardiac surgery. Moreover, patients with acute respiratory failure will be given glucocorticoids, nitric oxide, ketoconazole, N-acetylcysteine and a whole range of therapies with cursory consideration of the results, and ignoring the exclusion criteria, appearing to support their use.

To convert the reported benefit of any trial to something that is relevant to clinical practice, the clinician must assess the similarity of his or her untreated patient to the control group described, so that the likelihood of effectiveness of therapy can be judged appropriately.[3,4] It is often forgotten that there are many criteria within the report that may have excluded the patient from the trial in the first place, and thus exclude the conclusions reached being valid for the clinician's patient. Blind application of the results of any clinical study can be hazardous, as there are usually good reasons why a particular study excludes patients from the 'treatment' group in the first place. For example, previous studies may have found the treatment to be of no use, or even dangerous in the 'excluded' group of patients.

There is no substitute for thinking. When managing a patient with an acute clinical problem, an intelligent and alert practitioner is always required.[5]

REFERENCES
1. Packer M, Coats AJ, Fowler MB, et al. Effect of carvedilol on survival in severe chronic heart failure. N Engl J Med 2001;344:1651-1658.
2. Hébert PC, Wells G, Blajchman MA, Marshall J, Martin C, Pagliarello G , et al. A multicenter, randomised, controlled clinical trial of transfusion requirements in critical care. N Engl J Med 1999;340:409-417.

3. Sackett DL Haynes RB. Summarising the effects of therapy: a new table and some more terms. Evidence-based Medicine 1997;2:103-104.
4. Sackett DL, Richardson WS, Rosenberg W, Haynes RB. Evidence-based medicine. How to practice & teach EBM. Edinburgh: Churchill Livingstone. 1997.
5. Naylor CD. Clinical decisions: from art to science and back again. Lancet 2001;358(9281):523-524.

God heals and the doctor takes the fee

*"I work all night, I work all day, to pay the bills I have to pay.
Ain't it sad
And still it never seems to be a single penny left for me.
That's too bad"*
 ABBA

For the first 24 years following my graduation I worked in two major public teaching hospitals, first as a trainee medical specialist at the Queen Elizabeth Hospital, then as a specialist in anaesthesia and intensive care at the Royal Adelaide Hospital. Eight years after receiving my first pay cheque, my wife and I were finally able to convince a bank to lend us some money to build a house on the outskirts of Adelaide. I remained a public servant for the next sixteen years. When I left the Royal Adelaide Hospital to work at the Flinders Medical Centre, I still had a mortgage and responsibility for maintaining my last child through his final two years of tertiary education.

Up until that point I had spent most of my working life concerned with no other matter other than providing safe, effective and timely acute medical care to public ICU patients. I had very little private practice. However, as the Flinders Medical Centre intensivists serviced three private intensive care units as well as a large public ICU, part of my responsibilities involved the servicing of this private practice. While I enjoyed my allocated time in managing these patients, I learnt many lessons.

Firstly, there were differences in the specialist's remuneration. In the public system, the specialist is paid a wage from the public purse unrelated to the number of patients or procedures that he or she performs. The patient is not directly invoiced for the service. In the private system the specialist invoices the patient for each service provided, which may be remunerated wholly by the medical benefits scheme (i.e. government rebate) or by the government rebate and a private insurer. In both cases the patient may not be invoiced directly,

L. I. G. Worthley

but will be advised of the cost. If the rebate and insured difference does not cover the invoice fully, the difference – or gap – is paid by the patient, who should have agreed to this arrangement previously.

Secondly, I have found that if you discuss your income with anybody, for example colleagues or friends, it is likely that your wage will be thought of as excessive. H. L. Mencken describes a wealthy man as one "who earns $100 a year more than his wife's sister's husband", so I knew I was on a hiding-to-nothing when trying to reason with one of my patient's daughters concerning my account to her father.

"Dear Sir," her letter began. "My father was admitted to the Flinders Private Hospital late last year with a severe pneumonia needing life support for twenty three days in the intensive care unit. Thankfully, he survived and our family is grateful for the attention and care he received during this episode.

However, we have just received your account, which states that while medical benefits will pay most of his bill, he is required to pay an extra $558.50 as a 'gap' payment. As we were not informed of this prior to his admission and as he is a pensioner with minimal income, we believe that the extra amount is both unfair and wrong and are considering advising the South Australian Ombudsman about this matter. We would therefore ask you to please reconsider your account.

Yours sincerely"

As I was one of a group of intensive care specialists who saw this patient during his admission to the ICU, I was asked to reply to the letter on behalf of the group; which I did, without pleasure, by stating:

"Dear Mrs . . . .

Thank you for your letter of the 8.2.08. Our group of intensive care specialists strongly support a no-gap arrangement and as such have come to a mutually acceptable agreement with 43 health funds in this regard (I have enclosed a brochure listing the funds that have a 'no-gap' payment arrangement with us). However, while we have tried, a similar arrangement has not been reached with your fund.

Accordingly, they do not fully cover our services, which, in the case of your good father, were required when managing his life-threatening illness. Concerning prior consent to our services, we provided urgent intensive care treatment to your father in good faith after you had signed on his behalf the admission form that stated: "Should I require treatment by an intensivist, I may incur out-of-pocket expenses" (a copy of this form is included for your information).

We welcome the involvement of the Ombudsman and believe that you should also request in writing from your health care fund why they do not wish to provide, for their members, the mutually agreeable 'no gap' arrangement that we have reached with other health funds. Concerning the matter of the current gap payment for your father's account, could you please phone our accounts manager, as I am sure that a mutually acceptable solution can be reached.

Yours sincerely"

I phoned our accounts manager and told her to expect a phone call from the patient's daughter and asked her to please waive the requirement for the 'gap' payment.

I must say that I was genuinely troubled by this episode and continued to think about it for some time. Essentially, the viability of any business, and a medical partnership is a business, requires a profit to be made. If the business makes a loss and continues to do so, it will fail. While most medical groups have a manager to run their business and these businesses are rarely, if ever, unprofitable, the clinician is usually oblivious to matters such as cash flow, expenses, assets, liabilities, etc. Moreover, if a doctor considers the issue of making money as an essential focus of his or her practice, they will soon make this focus the primary goal, and the care of their patients will suffer.

Trust in one's physician is an essential but fragile element of good medical care.[1] Accordingly, to maintain trust, discussions pertaining to fee-for-service must be with the clear understanding that the doctor's responsibility to the patient will always take precedence over the clinician's economic self interest. The doctor should be a trustee not a provider and the patient should be a beneficiary not a customer.

REFERENCES
1. Relman AS. Doctors and the dispensing of drugs. N Engl J Med 1987;317:311-312.

Protocols without thought are dangerous

"A foolish consistency is the hobgoblin of little minds, adored by little statesmen and philosophers and divines."
Ralph Waldo Emerson

Protocols that guide the delivery of drugs are often employed in the management of critically ill patients. For example, protocols are often used in the ICU for drug infusions that control sedation or pain relief in the mechanically ventilated patient, blood pressure in the hypo- or hypertensive patient, and glycaemia in the diabetic patient. However, the patient still needs to be monitored carefully as treatment outside protocol guidelines may be required in the unstable patient.

A 24 year-old woman was admitted to hospital with a 'resistant' asthma attack. She had a past history of mild asthma since childhood, which could be exacerbated by upper respiratory tract infections, exercise and red wine. She had been admitted for severe asthma on four occasions previously, although for the last two years she had been well controlled on budesonide 200 µg 12-hourly and intermittent use of a salbutamol inhaler.

On her current admission she had a 12 hr history of progressive shortness of breath and persistent cough following a recent sore throat. Her salbutamol inhaler had given her some relief, but it had not been sustained. In the A&E department her pulse was 120 beats per minute, respiratory rate 28 per minute, temperature 36.8°C and on auscultation she had generalised wheezing. Her chest X-ray showed no major abnormality apart from moderate hyperinflation. Her arterial blood gas analysis revealed a PaO_2 of 72 mmHg, $PaCO_2$ 31 mmHg and pH 7.43.

The standard protocol for an acute asthma attack in the A&E department required continuous nebulised salbutamol and intravenous hydrocortisone 100 mg 6-hourly. However in spite of treatment, throughout the next 8 hours she became progressively more breathless and agitated. Finally, the A&E doctor phoned the ICU resident and said that he was sending up a severe asthmatic patient to intensive care saying that she "probably needed to be intubated."

When she arrived in the ICU, her pulse rate was 180 beats per minute and respiratory rate was 40 per minute, however her lungs on auscultation were clear. Her plasma biochemistry results were within normal limits apart from a low potassium level of 2.6 mmol/L. The arterial blood gas performed at this stage revealed a PaO_2 142 mmHg, $PaCO_2$ 24 mmHg, pH 7.37, bicarbonate 13 mmol/L and a base excess (BE) -11 mEq/L. It appeared that the continuous salbutamol inhalation had turned one form of respiratory distress, that of asthma, into another form of respiratory distress, that of metabolic acidosis with hyperventilation.

While continuous nebulised salbutamol may be the treatment of choice for acute severe asthma requiring hospital admission,[1,2] it should be used until an adequate clinical response occurs or adverse effects (e.g. tachycardia, arrhythmias, tremor or lactic acidosis) limits further administration.[3] The patient had an arterial blood lactate level on admission to the A&E department of 1.5 mmol/L with a BE -3 mEq/L. However eight hours later, when she was admitted to the ICU, the arterial blood lactate level had increased to 8.4 mmol/L with the BE decreasing to -11 mEq/L. The increasing breathlessness and agitation recorded by the A&E medical staff were erroneously considered to be due to a worsening of her asthmatic condition.

Hyperlactataemia has been linked to salbutamol therapy in asthma,[5] although lactic acidosis causing increasing breathlessness in the asthmatic patient has only been recorded infrequently.[4,5,6] While breathlessness may be due to worsening of the underlying asthma, requiring further bronchodilator therapy or even mechanical ventilation, lactic acidosis induced by salbutamol requires only discontinuation of salbutamol therapy.

Protocols have an important role to play in the management of an acutely ill patient. Nevertheless, continuous clinical assessment is mandatory during their use so that therapy can be discontinued when not required or when adverse effects occur.

REFERENCES
1. Olshaker J, Jerrard D, Barish RA, Brandt G, Hooper F. The efficacy and safety of a continuous albuterol protocol for the trteatment of acute adult asthma attacks. Am J Emerg Med 1993;11:131-133.
2. Calacone A, Wolkove N, Stern E, et al. Continuous nebulization of albuterol in acute asthma. Chest 1990;97:693-697.
3. Hegde RM, Worthley LIG. Acute asthma and the life threatening episode. Crit Care Resusc 1999;1:371-387.
4. Maury E, Ioos V, Lepecq B, Guidet B, Offenstadt G. A paradoxical effect of bronchodilators. Chest 1997;111:1766-1767.
5. Assadi FK. Therapy of acute bronchospasm. Complicated by lactic acidosis and hypokalemia. Clin Pediatr 1989;28:258-260.
6. Guichenez P, Girard-Madoux MH, Coppere B, Sanson C, Ninet J. Metabolic acidosis related to salbutamol use during treatment of acute bronchospasm. Rev Pneumol Clin 1991;47:270.

"Ill be there in a minute"

"Begin at the beginning," the King said gravely, "and go on till you come to the end: then stop."
Lewis Carroll

In Australia, admission to and discharge from an intensive care unit is the responsibility of the intensive care specialist – no one else. Nevertheless, many of my medical colleagues tend to forget this as they often phone with an indolent request of: "I want a patient to be admitted to intensive care." As I grew older I became less troubled with such requests, and rather than remind them of the admission and discharge policies of the unit, I would just listen to the story.

From the history outlined by the requesting specialist, I would gauge whether the clinician wanted my opinion concerning the diagnosis and severity of the patient's condition, or just wanted to reduce his or her responsibility for the patient by admitting them to an ICU bed. I would then try to determine how the patient would benefit from an intensive care admission. For example, if the patient was critically ill with a reversible life-threatening illness, ICU admission would be required. However, if the patient was 'not for resuscitation' – the admission would seem to be futile; if the patient's vital signs did not met the criteria for a medical emergency team (MET) call – unless the patient was unstable, the admission would seem to be unnecessary; and if the patient needed an emergency operation (e.g. for a ruptured aneurysm) – delaying the operation by admitting the patient to the ICU, rather than to the operating theatre, would seem to be unhelpful. But before I made a determination I would usually see the patient, to make my own assessment as to what benefit an ICU admission would be and how I could help.

If a request 'for ICU admission' was received during the working day the patient would be somewhere within the hospital so it would be easy for me to see them and determine the nature of the problem. However, if I were at home and asleep my approach would be simplified. I would determine whether I needed to get dressed and come in to review the patient, or whether I could admit the patient to the ICU under the care of the resident ICU doctor who would then keep me informed of any critical change. I would see the patient in the morning. Fortunately the hospitals that I serviced were no more than 15 minutes away so, more often than not, I would dress and drive in to review the patient.

As soon as I made up my mind that I needed to come in, and this was usually determined within a minute or so, I would say, without further questioning, "I'll be there in a minute."

One such nocturnal episode occurred late in my career at one of the private hospitals, and began with a phone call from the A&E resident:

"Dr. Worthley, I have an 82 year old man who was brought in by the ambulance one hour ago. He has a sharp stabbing pain in his upper left thigh, a pain that is relatively short in duration and intermittent, although sometimes it is more prolonged, and of a dull nature. If the pain radiates to his right side his blood pressure falls from 120 mmHg systolic to 90 mmHg systolic and this is associated with a slowing of his AF which developed in the last 30 minutes, with no change in his ECG . . . ."

I made my mind up early in his presentation that I needed to come in to see the patient, as I had no idea from the A&E resident's history what was happening. However, as he babbled on without taking a breath, I could not terminate the conversation with my well worn "I'll be there in a minute." My wife was awake at this point and as I had not said anything for some time, I think she thought I had gone back to sleep. After a while I needed to go to the bathroom, so I put the receiver on the pillow and got up.

"What are you doing?" asked my wife.

"I'm going to have a pee," I said, and in the darkness moved toward our *en suite* toilet.

"But what about the phone call?" she said.

"He's still talking. He won't notice I've gone."

"But . . . " She gave up as I closed the toilet door.

It would have been at least one or two minutes later that I returned to pick up the phone. The registrar was still talking. Finally he said "what do you want me to do?"

"I'll be there in a minute." I said, hung up and began to dress.

Should the replacement of acute blood loss with non-red blood cell solutions in the elderly be called resuscitation or embalming?

"... *bloodletting is intertwined in the mysterious fabric of medical lore; it originated from magic and religious ceremonies. The physician and priest were one and the same since disease was thought to be caused by supernatural causes."*
Gilbert R. Seigworth

Mr Wellington was an 84 year old man who had a past history of hypertension, ischaemic heart disease and chronic bronchitis. He had just been admitted to the intensive care unit following an elective repair of an abdominal aortic aneurysm. He was pale, with low blood pressure and in severe pulmonary oedema with the anaesthetic registrar beginning the 'hand over' as he struggled to position the bed into the bay.

It appeared that the operation was technically complicated. However, no blood had been given throughout the procedure even though an assessed blood loss of 4 litres was recorded. Instead, 3 litres of 4% albumin in 0.9% saline, 3 litres of Gelofusine® and 6 litres of Hartmann's solution were administered "for intravascular loading" and to replace the "volume loss". During our conversation it also emerged that at the latter part of the 3-hour operation the patient's cardiac monitor revealed "sagging" of the ST segments, so he was given atenolol "15 mg all up" but then developed hypotension requiring intermittent metaraminol during the final stage of the operation. As the pulse oximeter recorded an ever-decreasing saturation, the inspired oxygen concentration was gradually increased from 40% to 100%, with positive end expiratory pressure being finally applied to stop the blood-stained froth from entering the expiratory limb of the

71

anaesthetic circuit. A blood gas, which was performed just before leaving the operating theatre, suddenly appeared and revealed a PaO_2 65 mmHg, $PaCO_2$ 57 mmHg, pH 7.01, lactate 9 mmol/L and haemoglobin 61 g/L.

"You didn't use blood because . . . ?" I left a pause for the anaesthetic registrar to reply.

"We are not using blood routinely," he said "ever since the Canadian study showed that it increases mortality."

"Increases mortality!" I uttered.

"Yeah, it increases mortality if used routinely," he blurted.

I could not help myself. "But he is now in cardiogenic shock and severe pulmonary oedema. In fact, I can't think of anything else you could have done that would have made his condition worse. He was generously preloaded, his haemoglobin has more than halved, with resultant cardiac ischaemia; he was then beta-blocked, reducing inotropism, and the metaraminol selectively increased his afterload, increasing cardiac work and left atrial pressure. Voilà! - cardiogenic shock and fulminant pulmonary oedema!"

His chin protruded. "OK, what would you have done?"

"I would have given blood – the other problems would not have occurred."

He put his metaraminol syringe into his top pocket, looked at me for a second and smirked. "Enjoy," he said, then turned and left, leaving me to regret my outburst.

'Blood and blood products are a limited resource and should be used within strict guidelines' is a statement that has no rebuttal and every major hospital will have their protocols for transfusion. However many confuse the indications for a red blood cell (RBC) transfusion in the elderly patient who is acutely anaemic (e.g. during resuscitation for active haemorrhage) for those indications that are based on studies performed in normovolaemic patients with chronic anaemia.

Fundamentally, the equation is relatively simple. Life cannot exist in humans without red blood cells and the closer we get to this point, the greater we jeopardise life. Nevertheless a red blood cell transfusion is not risk free and is indicated when its benefit, i.e. to sustain life, is greater than its risk, i.e. to threaten life.

In a young and healthy human, the haemoglobin ranges between 130 – 180 g/L in males and 120 – 160 g/L in females. An acute normovolaemic reduction of haemoglobin to 50 g/L does not produce evidence of inadequate systemic oxygen delivery, as assessed by a rise in arterial blood lactate or ST segment changes in the electrocardiogram.[1] The minimal haemoglobin level required in the absence of disease and at rest is 30 g/L.[1] Indeed, a patient who survived with maximum cardiovascular and respiratory support with a haemoglobin level of 14 g/L has been recorded.[2] Nonetheless in the elderly patient with co-morbid conditions that include ischaemic cardiac disease, an acute isovolaemic reduction in RBC mass can produce profound effects, as their ability to increase cardiac output and to selectively vasodilate threatened organs to improve oxygen supply is often severely limited.

In a study by the 'TRICC' investigators of 4470 critically ill patients, anaemia (i.e. haemoglobin < 100 g/L) was associated with an increased risk of death in patients with cardiac disease, and that blood transfusions decreased this risk.[3] Yet a multicentre randomised trial of 838 critically ill anaemic patients reported by the same group, found a restrictive transfusion approach (i.e. one that kept the haemoglobin between 70 - 90 g/L) was just as effective, and was associated with a lower mortality rate, compared to a liberal transfusion approach (i.e. one that kept the haemoglobin between 100 - 120 g/L).[4] Nevertheless these investigators retrospectively reviewed a subgroup of 357 patients who were anaemic with a diagnosis of coronary artery disease from their study of 836 critically ill patients,[4] and reported a trend to a lower survival rate in the group with a restrictive transfusion approach compared with the liberal transfusion group.[5]

A relationship between mortality and anaemia has been established in elderly patients with cardiovascular disease.[6,7] In one retrospective study of 78974 patients who were ≥ 65 years old and who were admitted to hospital with acute myocardial infarction, blood transfusion was associated with a lower 30 day mortality in patients who had a haematocrit on admission less than 33% (i.e. 110 g/L).[8]

Also, in a randomised trial of patients with congestive heart failure, an increase in the haemoglobin from 103 g/L to 129 g/L was associated with an improved left ventricular ejection fraction and a reduction in diuretic dose compared with the control group. During the study, the treatment group had no mortality compared with the control group, which had a mortality of 25%.[9]

Nonetheless, in an observational study of three large randomised trials involving 24111 patients who had an acute myocardial infarct, Rao *et al*, using sophisticated analytic methods and in a younger group of patients, concluded that transfusion, which occurred in only 10% of patients, may have increased mortality.[10] Moreover, a recent study of 2016 patients who were ≥ 50 years old, who had either a history of, or risk factors for, cardiovascular disease, and whose haemoglobin level was below 100 g/L after hip-fracture surgery, found that a liberal transfusion strategy (i.e. to transfuse if the haemoglobin level > 10 g/L) did not reduce the 60 day mortality rate when compared with patients who had a restrictive transfusion strategy (i.e. to transfuse if the haemoglobin level was < 80 g/L).[11] However, both studies were concerned with patients who were stable and not actively bleeding. Furthermore, transfusions in the latter study for 'symptoms' occurred more often in the restrictive strategy group, and protocol violations resulting in additional transfusions may have altered the mortality in this group.[12]

In patients with chronic kidney disease and chronic anaemia, relationships between anaemia, morbidity[13,14] and mortality[15,16] have been reported, leading to guidelines that recommend blood haemoglobin be maintained between 110 g/L and 120 g/L in these patients.[17]

Apart from the mechanical effects (e.g. air embolism, micro-embolism, hypervolaemia) and febrile reactions, which are rarely life-threatening,[18] the risks associated with RBC transfusions include haemolytic reactions which may be life-threatening when incompatible RBCs are administered,[19] anaphylactoid reactions,[20] disease transmission (while blood is normally screened, infections may be still be transmitted with an incidence of 1:5,000,000 for HIV, 1:3,000,000 for HCV and 1:1,000,000 for HBV) and bacterial infections. However, of

Inside God's Shed

the proposed transfusion-related immunomodulation (TRIM) effects, which include improved renal allograft survival,[21,22] enhancement of metastatic spread of carcinoma,[23,24,25] increase in postoperative infectious complications[24,26] and graft vs. host disease, improved renal allograft survival is the only TRIM effect that has been demonstrated unequivocally at the clinical level.[21,22,24,27,28]

Traditionally, a haemoglobin level of 100 g/L in a normovolaemic patient has been taken as the value below which a transfusion is required, although a single threshold for transfusion applied to all patients is a coarse reference.[29] Current data suggest that the threshold should probably be at a haemoglobin level < 80 g/L in the young patient and < 100 g/L in the elderly patient with active cardiovascular disease.[20,30,31,32,33,34,35,36] In the actively bleeding patient the use of non-RBC fluid rather than RBCs is well tolerated in the healthy young patient, as they can endure a normovolaemic drop in haemoglobin by up to 70%. However in the elderly patient (e.g. ≥ 65 years old) with cardiovascular co-morbid conditions, any acute drop in haemoglobin can be hazardous and deliberate normovolaemic resuscitation using non-RBC fluid rather than RBC in this group may reflect more a process of embalming rather than resuscitation.

REFERENCES
1. Weiskopf RB, Viele MK, Feiner J, Kelley S, Lieberman J, Noorani M, et al. Human cardiovascular and metabolic response to acute, severe isovolemic anemia. JAMA 1998;279:217-221.
2. Brimacombe J, Skippen P, Talbutt P. Acute anaemia to a haemoglobin of 14 g.L-1 with survival. Anaesth Intens Care 1991;19:581-583.
3. Hébert PC, Wells G, Tweeddale M, Martin C, Marshall J, Pham B, et al, for the Transfusion Requirements in Critical Care (TRICC) Investigators and the Canadian Critical Care Trials Group. Does transfusion practice affect mortality in critically ill patients. Am J Resp Crit Care Med 1997;155:1618-1623.
4. Hébert PC, Wells G, Blajchman MA, Marshall J, Martin C, Pagliarello G, et al, and the Transfusion Requirements in Critical Care (TRICC) Investigators for the Canadian Critical Care Trials

Group. A multicenter, randomised, controlled clinical trial of transfusion requirements in critical care. N Engl J Med 1999;340:409-417.
5. Hébert PC, Yetisir E, Martin C, Blajchman MA, Wells G, Marshall J, et al, the Transfusion Requirements in Critical Care Investigators for the Canadian Critical Care Trials Group. Is a low transfusion threshold safe in critically ill patients with cardiovascular diseases? Crit Care Med 2001;29:227-234.
6. Lenfant C. Transfusion should be monitored for undertransfusion as well as overtransfusion. Transfusion 1992;32:873-874.
7. Sazama K. Is undertransfusion occuring? Transfusion 2001;41:577-578.
8. Wu W-C, Rathore SS, Wang Y, Radfpord MJ, Krumholz HM. Blood transfusion in elderly patients with acute myocardial infarction. N Engl J Med 2001;345:1230-1236.
9. Silverberg DS, Wexler D, Sheps D, Blum M, Keren G, Baruch R, et al. The effect of correction of mild anemia in severe, resistant congestive heart failure using subcutaneous erythropoietin and intravenous iron: a randomized controlled study. J Am Coll Cardiol 2001;37:1775-1780.
10. Rao SV, Jollis JG, Harrington RA, Granger CB, Newby LK, Armstrong PW, et al. Relationship of blood transfusion and clinical outcomes in patients with acute coronary syndromes. JAMA 2004;292:1555-1562.
11. Carson JL, Terrin ML, Noveck H, Sanders DW, Chaitman BR, Rhoads GG, et al, for the FOCUS Investigators. Liberal or restrictive transfusion in high-risk patients after hip surgery. N Engl J Med 2011;365:2453-2462.
12. Barr PJ, Bailie KEM. Transfusion thresholds in FOCUS. N Engl J Med 2011;365:2532-2533.
13. Besarab A, Bolton WK, Browne JK, Egrie JC, Nissenson AR, Okamoto DM, et al. The effects of normal as compared with low hematocrit values in patients with cardiac disease who are receiving hemodialysis and epoetin. N Engl J Med 1998;339:584-590.

14. Collins A, Ma JZ, Ebben J. Impact of hematocrit on morbidity and mortality. Semin Nephrol 2000;20:345-349.
15. Ma J, Ebben J, Xia H, Collins AJ. Hematocrit level and associated mortality in hemodialysis patients. J Am Soc Nephrol 1999;10:610-619.
16. Collins AJ, Li S, St Peter W, Ebben J, Roberts T, Ma JZ, et al. Death, hospitalization, and economic associations among incident hemodialysis patients with hematocrit values of 36 to 39%. J Am Soc Nephrol. 2001;12:2465-2473.
17. National Kidney Foundation. K/DOQL. Clinical practice guidelines for the treatment of anemia of chronic renal failure. Am J Kidney Dis 1997;30:S192-237.
18. Mollison PL. Blood transfusion in clinical medicine. Blackwell Scientific Publications, Oxford 1979.
19. Greenwalt TJ. Pathogenesis and management of hemolytic transfusion reactions. Seminars in Hematology 1981;18:84-94.
20. Carson JL, Duff A, Poses RM, Berlin JA, Spence RK, Trout R, et al. Effect of anaemia and cardiovascular disease on surgical mortality and morbidity. Lancet 1996;348 (9034):1055-1160.
21. Pereira A. Deleterious consequences of allogenic blood transfusion on postoperative infection: really a transfusion-related immunomodulation effect? Blood 2001;98:498-500.
22. Opelz G, Sengar DP, Mickey MR, Terasaki PI. Effect of blood transfusions on subsequent kidney transplants. Transplant Proc 1973;5:253-259.
23. Stephenson KR, Steinberg SM, Hughes KS, Vetto JT, Sugarbaker PH, Chang AE. Perioperative blood transfusions are associated with decreased time to recurrence and decreased survival after resection of colorectal liver metastases. Ann Surg 1988;208:679-687.
24. Vamvakas EC, Blajchman MA. Deleterious clinical effects of transfusion-associated immunomodulation: fact or fiction? Blood 2001;97:1180-1195.

25. Busch ORC, Hop WCJ, Hoynck van Papendrecht MAW, Marquet RL, Jeekel J. Blood transfusions and the prognosis of colorectal cancer. N Engl J Med 1993;328:1372-1376.
26. Heiss MM, Mempel W, Jauch K-W, Delanoff C, Mayer G, Mempel M, et al. Beneficial effect of autologous blood transfusion on infectious complications after colorectal cancer. Lancet 1993;342(8883):1328-1333.
27. Schriemer PA, Longnecker DE, Mintz PD. The possible immunosuppressive effects of perioperative blood transfusion in cancer patients. Anesthesiology 1988;68:422-428.
28. Sanfilippo F, Spees EK, Vaughn WK. The timing of pretransplant transfusions and renal allograft survival. Transplantation 1984;37:344-350.
29. Surgenor SD, Hampers MJ, Corwin HL. Is blood transfusion good for the heart? Crit Care Med 2001;29:442-444.
30. Goodnough LT, Brecher ME, Kanter MH, AuBuchon JP. Transfusion medicine – Blood transfusion. N Engl J Med 1999;340:438-447.
31. Hébert PC, Fergusson DA. Do transfusions get to the heart of the matter? JAMA 2004;292:1610-1612.
32. Practice guidelines for blood component therapy: a report by the American Society of Anesthesiologists Task force on Blood Component Therapy. Anesthesiology 1996;84:732-747.
33. Nicholls MD, Whyte G. Red cell, FFP and albumin transfusion triggers. Anaesth Intens Care 1993;21:156-162.
34. Consensus statement on red cell transfusion. Transfus Med 1994;4:177-178.
35. Cane RD. Hemoglobin: how much is enough? Crit Care Med 1990;18:1046.
36. Hogue CW Jr, Goodnough LT, Monk TG. Perioperative myocardial ischemic episodes are related to hematocrit level in patients undergoing radical prostatectomy. Transfusion 1998;38:924-931.

"Mr Smith would want to have the operation"

"Moral indignation is a technique used to endow the idiot with dignity."
Marshall McLuhan

We were at a meeting discussing the management of Mr. Smith, a 79 year old severely demented gentleman, and were trying to reach a consensus about the best treatment for his thoracic aortic aneurysm. He had no immediate family, his wife died some 6 years ago and while he had been living independently at home for the first few years after this, his neighbours soon discovered that he often put his rubbish bins out on the wrong day, continually wore the same clothes, and appeared to be losing weight. It soon became evident that he wasn't managing by himself. After many supportive services were called upon to help him at home, ultimately he needed to be admitted to a nursing home. A guardian was appointed and he soon became completely dependent for showering, dressing, toileting and eating. He spent most of his life sitting outside in a chair asleep, or inside in front of a TV asleep.

From his medical history, the guardian noted that he saw a doctor every three months to review his hypertension, peripheral vascular disease, ischaemic heart disease and mild renal failure. He had a coronary bypass procedure 4 years earlier and ever since that operation his local doctor believed that he had never really returned to his previous good health. The local doctor informed the guardian that the patient had a slowly expanding thoracic aneurysm that had recently caused some mild aortic regurgitation, and suggested that perhaps a review by a cardiothoracic surgeon may be in order.

Here we were: a cardiothoracic surgeon, an intensivist (me), an anaesthetist, the hospital deputy administrator, a geriatrician and the patient's guardian, all of whom were up to 15 years younger than me, assessing the benefits or otherwise of a major cardiothoracic operation

L. I. G. Worthley

– a Bentall procedure (i.e. replacement the ascending aorta and the aortic valve and reimplanting both coronary arteries into the graft), in this man.

"The mortality from a Bentall procedure is less than 3%, and the five year survival rate should be greater than 90%," said the surgeon when asked about the risk associated with the disease.

"Would the patient's age, underlying cardiovascular disease and dementia, make any difference to his prognosis?" I said hoping to get a more specific response from the surgeon.

"Maybe . . . maybe not," was his less than useful answer.

"What about the likelihood of living another 5 years if he just had cardiovascular disease, mild renal failure and severe dementia – but without the thoracic aneurysm?" I said, looking at the geriatrician.

"He could possibly live another 5 years," was the answer that was equally unhelpful.

"And that's very likely?" I continued.

"Oh . . . its likely," the geriatrician mused.

I started to doodle. I've found it soothed me at meetings that drifted into 'decision oblivion'.

"Well then," said the deputy administrator, who was chairing the meeting.

"It seems that the operation might be of benefit then?"

There was silence.

I felt that the meeting could not just end there with some 'wooden' statistics for the guardian to make a judgement, so I finally said, "as far as the postoperative course for this man in the intensive care unit is concerned, I can see a very likely scenario of a prolonged episode of acute respiratory failure. He is severely demented and would be uncooperative with coughing and breathing exercises, thereby retaining sputum and requiring a tracheotomy for further management. His mild renal failure would worsen and need dialysis if severe, and Mr. Smith would be put through an enormous amount of pain and distress without adding any more years to his life."

Again there was silence.

"So you don't believe he deserves an operation then?" said the guardian who had been silent up to this point.

Inside God's Shed

"It is not a question of deserving, it is a question of what would be the best option for him so that he could enjoy whatever life he has left, free of pain, comfortable and in no distress," I said, wishing that I had continued to doodle as I knew where this meeting was heading.

She politely listened to me then said, "As the patient's guardian, it is up to me to determine what he would and would not want, and in listening to you all I am sure that Mr. Smith would want to have the operation."

I wasn't surprised. The wrong decision had been made apparently for the right political reasons. We wouldn't want to see on the front page of the local newspaper the headlines, 'Nursing home patient denied life-saving operation'.

The patient's needs should have been 'front and centre'. Instead, some at the meeting were more interested in covering their own backsides, in case of political fallout. We occasionally admit patients to the intensive care unit after a cardiac arrest, who unfortunately progress to a vegetative state due to irreversible brain damage. If a guardian has been involved, full resuscitative measures and tracheostomy are often recommended because they deem 'the patient would want it', saying that to do otherwise would be to consider the policies of Nazi Germany in the management of disabled patients.

If our society is judged by how we treat our infirm patients, we should insure that the treatment provided is the best we can achieve for the underlying medical condition, without any influence of the perceived 'value of a life'. When considering the differences between medical and surgical management for a disorder, medical treatment does not mean 'no' treatment and surgical treatment does not mean 'best' treatment.

What happened to Mr. Smith? He underwent the operation and died in theatre.

Spare me the pain

"All substances are poisons; there is none which is not a poison. The right dose differentiates a poison and a remedy."
Paracelsus

In many public hospitals a chronic pain clinic exists to deal with the complex nature of the body's response to injury, particularly in patients who have a chronic or terminal illness. These clinics are indispensable, although their waiting lists are often brutally long with few well-trained specialists able to meet the clinical demand.[1] An acute pain service may also exist, particularly if the hospital has a busy surgical service, as surgeons are usually in theatre and postoperative pain is often managed poorly by a routine order given to the nursing staff. Treatment of pain in these patients is managed more effectively by a group of specialists who 'round' daily or twice daily to individualise therapy. These acute pain specialists have their own training and accreditation programs, their own journals and scientific meetings.

However, and particularly early in the development of this service, there were occasional difficulties in the dual management of pain in the acutely ill patient when both the intensivist and pain medicine specialist were involved. Acutely ill patients in ICU are monitored closely and if their condition deteriorates, therapy may need to be changed immediately. To prescribe a standard opiate infusion for pain, to be reviewed some time later, in a critically ill patient is usually fraught with danger. Moreover, pain is a symptom, so the cause should be diagnosed before treatment is prescribed. In an acutely ill postoperative abdominal surgical patient, pain can be caused by conditions other than surgical injury, including an obstructed, infarcted or perforated bowel. The patient should be carefully assessed before pain relief is prescribed.

Some time ago, a postoperative abdominal aortic aneurysm patient was admitted to the high dependency unit (HDU) for acute pain management by the acute pain clinic. A morphine infusion was ordered with the nurse instructed to increase the infusion if the patient had any pain. The nurse dutifully followed the orders and asked the patient had he any pain, increasing the morphine dose every time the patient responded with a "yes". Over the course of the day the patient soon had to be woken to answer the question, although the patient's answer remained the same. Later that afternoon, the ICU registrar was called to an emergency in the HDU when the patient was found to be unconscious and 'gurgling'. The patient was intubated, without an anaesthetic, the morphine was discontinued and following tracheal suctioning, fluid administration, a small dose of adrenaline and prophylactic antibiotic administration, he was admitted to the ICU.

"Who discontinued the morphine?" was the response of the acute pain specialist when she reviewed the patient in ICU.

"I did. He was being permanently anaesthetised," I said in an effort to take the conversation to a sudden halt.

"Rubbish!" was her reply, "the patient is still in pain."

"The patient is unconscious!" I retorted. "Your morphine infusions overdose patients. Patients will always say, "yes" to the question 'do you have any pain?' You should ask them 'are you comfortable?' because they want comfort not anaesthesia."

I then added my usual provocation, "the fundamental fact is - pain never killed anybody but pain relief has."

She remained silent for a second, so I enquired, "how many patients have you seen die due to pain?"

"Pain provokes a severe sympathetic response and in a patient who has critical ischaemic heart disease there is likely, more often than not...."

I interrupted, "so you've seen no one die of pain?"

I was building to a crescendo.

"You see, if pain was such a lethal condition, the human race would not have survived – we would have died out long ago with the massive death rate associated with pain of childbirth!"

"You, of course, know what it's like to have labour pain," she said injecting a large piece of sarcasm.

I ignored the comment and added, "only nerve blocks or obliteration of the nerve pathway will completely relieve pain, the opiate infusion will only completely relieve pain if the patient is unconscious."

She turned and left, thereafter avoiding me.

To be fair, this episode occurred early in the development of the acute pain service at our hospital. Techniques that include patient controlled analgesia and specialised spinal analgesia, to mention but two useful ways to manage acute postoperative pain, have been developed by the specialty to allow safe and effective methods to treat pain, even in the acutely ill patient.

REFERENCES
1. Pizzo PA, Clark NM. Alleviating suffering 101 – pain relief in the United States. N Engl J Med 2012;366:197-199.

Cardiac arrest teams, medical emergency teams and rapid-response teams. Are we going backwards?

"God punishes us mildly by ignoring our prayers and severely by answering them."
Richard J. Needham

Monday morning ward round at the public hospital ICU when I was first 'on call' – how I dreaded it. I often arrived one hour early to do a quick uninterrupted patient review to get a feeling of who were sick, and really needed help, and who were not (e.g. were eating breakfast while looking at the overhead TV). The latter were often admitted to ICU because they had triggered one of the non-specific medical emergency team (MET) criteria in the general wards over the weekend. As the home clinic were unable to be contacted, or were unwilling to take responsibility for the patient, the patient would be admitted to the ICU. When I questioned the benefits of this system, some of my ICU colleagues would say,

"Don't you think that the patient is better off being treated by us than managed in the ward?" to which I would reply,

"With that logic, why don't we manage the whole hospital?"

Some would retort without expecting a reply "perhaps we should."

The MET system had only recently been introduced at our hospital. Previously, when a cardiac arrest, respiratory arrest or seizure occurred, or a patient became unconscious in a general hospital ward, a 'cardiac arrest team' provided immediate resuscitation. However, as some studies suggested that up to 88% of in-hospital cardiac arrests were preceded by at least one abnormal clinical feature[1,2,3,4,5] a MET to respond to these abnormalities was proposed to reduce the in-hospital mortality.[6] The medical emergency team consisted of clinicians who were paged to respond immediately to patients who had predefined abnormal observations that included: pulse < 40 or > 130 beats per

85

minute, respiration rate < 8 or > 30 breaths per minute, systolic blood pressure < 90 mmHg, pulse oximetry < 90%, urine output < 50 mL in 4 hours, change in conscious state or staff member was worried about the patient. As several studies reported a significant decrease in the incidence of cardiac arrests, unplanned intensive care admissions, and mortality rates when using these medical emergency teams, many hospitals embraced the concept enthusiastically and established a MET service, even though the early studies were not prospective, randomised or controlled.[7,8 9,10,11]

As I saw it, there were three problems with this new system, all of which impinged on patient care.

Firstly, the care of the patient who triggered the MET call could be compromised. For instance, in the case of a postoperative patient, if a crisis occurred and the surgeon was unavailable, the intensivist would manage the patient without the surgeon's advice. Accordingly, the possibility of a surgical reason for the emergency (e.g. bleeding, perforation, infarction) may be overlooked; a particular problem if the complication is hidden within the abdomen, chest or head – more on that later.

Secondly, the care of other ICU patients could be compromised as all ICU patients require a thorough review by the intensivist to exclude any pernicious problem before they are discharged, which takes time. Over the weekend up to 10 patients in a busy 40 bed ICU may be inappropriately admitted and could take the intensivist's attention away from patients who were sick and genuinely needed a specialist's consideration.[12]

Thirdly, the care of other inpatients who became critically ill could be compromised as there was often an 'exit block' when attempting to discharge inappropriately admitted patients to their home ward. Surgical waiting list patients or emergency department patients would rapidly fill the empty hospital beds. If the ICU was full, no one could be admitted ('we are full' – an entry block), and if the hospital was full no one could be discharged ('they are full' – an exit block). The ICU team would be responsible for the patients who remained, managing all non-life threatening problems. Any additional acutely ill patient would be queued in the A&E department or outlying general wards and would receive inadequate care.

Ultimately, a prospective randomised controlled study of the MET system was performed, which examined its effect on morbidity and mortality. It concluded with the statement "The MET system greatly increases emergency team calling, but does not substantially affect the incidence of cardiac arrest, unplanned ICU admissions, or unexpected death."[13] Two subsequent meta-analyses also failed to show a decrease in the rate of cardiac arrests in association with this new rapid-response system,[14,15] leading reviewers to conclude that "the effectiveness of such systems remains uncertain and a matter of controversy."[1]

Returning to the problem of the possibility of a compromise in the care of the patient who triggered the MET call, in a perverse irony, Dr. Buist, one of the protagonists of the MET system,[5,7,16] found himself a victim of this very fault, saying in a televised interview:[17]

"Last year in October I realised that I had appendicitis, so I was optimistic that this was going to be a quick and straightforward medical issue and that I'd be back on deck pretty quickly. But the following morning I felt absolutely dreadful. I called the nurse in because I just felt light-headed and she took my blood pressure and it was 60 millimetres of mercury. And she did absolutely the right thing. She called the medical emergency team. And here am I lying in bed thinking I've done all this fantastic research on medical emergency teams and I could see the irony of the situation that here it's coming to see me and save me. And then they did an electrocardiograph, an ECG, and that suggested quite strongly that I was having a heart attack. I said, "I am not having a heart attack. I don't have chest pain." But the medical emergency team doctor said to me, "Now look, you just lie there, you be the good patient. I'm in charge here, look at this ECG, you are not telling me that this is not a heart attack that you're having Mr. Intensive Care Specialist. You just be the patient." I had this overwhelming fear that I was going to die . . . and said, "Look, get the surgeon, I am bleeding." And the staff came up to me said, "No, there, there. You're okay. Your lips still look really pink and you're fine." And then I had to say, "Get the f***ing surgeon, I am bleeding."

Ultimately Dr. Buist's brother phoned the surgeon who re-operated and stopped the bleeding. Even his brother commented "You realise there's a huge irony in all of this. In some respects Michael almost got killed by his own invention."

This, along with other problems, were also highlighted in an editorial that concluded, "The problems facing MET are inappropriate management because the team is unfamiliar with the patient, inadequate staff level on wards, diversion of MET doctors away from their usual duties and conflict with the primary medical team. The evidence for the current model of MET is weak."[18]

On reflecting upon this event Dr. Buist stated that the episode "gave me the idea of . . . an ICT (information and communications technology) system where patient data is collected electronically . . . and automatically communicates abnormal patient results to the most appropriate health care provider"[17] (e.g. the surgeon).

To improve the MET response, the data that initiate a MET call (the afferent limb) should be modified so that if a response is initiated because 'a staff member is worried about the patient', the clinician responsible for the patient is contacted first and immediately. Mobile phones, even using an ICT system that Dr. Buist proposes, perhaps an 'app', could be useful in this regard. If the patient is suddenly unconscious, fitting, not breathing or pulseless this should initiate an immediate MET call (the efferent limb) and following resuscitation, the clinician responsible for the patient is contacted. To combat the second and third problems, the MET system must have sufficient resources (e.g. adequate staffing of the ICU) to provide ample care for all ICU patients, and appropriate discharge arrangements, to counter the problem of 'exit block'. These changes will ensure that an emergency medical team will be used appropriately and ICU's and their services will be employed effectively and efficiently.

Finally, an increase in DNR (do not resuscitate) and 'comfort care only' orders that followed the implementation of a MET system, in some studies, is of interest.[19,20] These orders should be made with due consultation with the patient, their relatives and clinician responsible for the patient, and made long before a MET call. Ideally, these orders should not be made at the patient's bedside whilst the team considers

Inside God's Shed

'for active resuscitation' or not, particularly if the team is headed by someone who has difficulty in diagnosing between an acute myocardial infarction and blood loss.[17]

REFERENCES
1. Jones DA, DeVita MA, Bellomo R. Rapid-response teams. N Engl J Med 2011;365:139-146.
2. Hillman KM, Bristow PJ, Chey T, Daffurn K, Jacques T, Norman SL, et al. Antecedents to hospital deaths. Intern Med J 2001;31:343-348.
3. Schein RM, Hazdat N, Pena M, Ruben BH, Sprung CL. Clinical antecedents to in-hospital-cardiopulmonary arrest. Chest 1990;98:1388-1392.
4. Franklin C, Mathew J. Developing strategies to prevent in-hospital cardiac arrest: Analyzing responses of physicians and nurses in the hours before the event. Crit Care Med 1994; 22:244-247.
5. Buist MD, Jarmolowski E, Burton PR, Bernard SA, Waxman BP, Anderson J. Recognising clinical instability in hospital patients before cardiac arrest or unplanned intensive care admission: A pilot study in a tertiary-care hospital. Med J Aust 1999;171:22-25.
6. Lee A, Bishop G, Hillman K, Daffurn K. The Medical Emergency Team. Anaesth Intensive Care 1995;23:183-186.
7. Buist MD, Moore GE, Bernard SA, Waxman BP, Anderson JN, Nguyen TV. Effects of a medical emergency team on reduction of incidence of and mortality from unexpected cardiac arrests in hospital: preliminary study. BMJ 2002;324:387-390.
8. Bellomo R, Goldsmith D, Uchino S, Buckmaster J, Hart GK, Opdam H, et al. A prospective before-and-after trial of a medical emergency team. Med J Aust 2003;179:283-288.
9. Ball C, Kirkby M, Williams S. Effect of the critical care outreach team on patient survival to discharge from hospital and readmission to critical care: non-randomised population based study. BMJ 2003;327:1014.
10. Bellomo R, Goldsmith D, Uchino S, Buckmaster J, Hart GK, Opdam H, et al. Prospective controlled trial of effect of medical

emergency team on postoperative morbidity and mortality rates. Crit Care Med 2004;32:916-921.
11. DeVita MA, Braithwaite R S, Mahidhara R, Stuart S, Foraida M, Simmons R L. Use of medical emergency team responses to reduce hospital cardiopulmonary arrests. Qual Saf Health Care 2004;13:251-254.
12. Winters BD, Pham J, Pronovost PJ. Rapid response teams — walk, don't run. JAMA 2006;296:1645-1647.
13. Hillman K, Chen J, Cretikos M, Bellomo R, Brown D, Doig G, et al; MERIT study investigators. Introduction of the medical emergency team (MET) system: a cluster-randomised controlled trial. Lancet 2005;365(9477):2091-2097.
14. Chan PS, Jain R, Nallmothu BK, Berg RA, Sasson C. Rapid response teams: a systematic review and meta-analysis. Arch Intern Med 2010;170:18-26.
15. McGaughey J, Alderdice F, Fowler R, Kapila A, Mayhew A, Moutray M. Outreach and early warning systems (EWS) for the prevention of intensive care admission and death of critically ill adult patients on general hospital wards. Cochrane Database Syst Rev 2007;3:CD005529.
16. Buist M, Bernard S, Nguyen T V, Moore G, Anderson J. Association between clinically abnormal observations and subsequent in-hospital mortality: A prospective study. Resuscitation 2004;62:137-141.
17. Australian Story "Doctor in the house" Monday 27th July 2009 http://www.abc.net.au/austory/content/2007/s2638546.htm (accessed April 2012).
18. Joyce C, McArthur C. Rapid response systems: have we MET the need? Crit Care Resusc 2007;9:127-128.
19. Felner K, Smith RL. Rapid-response teams. N Engl J Med 2011;365:1355.356.
20. Manthous CA. Rapid-response teams. N Engl J Med 2011;365:1356.

"... are you happy about that?"

"When doctors listen to nurses, patients recover more quickly."
Reg Revans

Change occurs everywhere, and no more so than in the intensive care unit. Technology has allowed monitoring to become unobtrusive and deceptively modest. Patients may be haemofiltered, dialysed, plasmapheresed, intra-aortic balloon counterpulsed, and ventilated in any level three intensive care unit bed without causing so much as a turn of an eye. The intensive care nurse has also undergone change, although I don't think that it would be described as unobtrusive. While they, as always, remain pivotal to the standard of care that is delivered by any intensive care unit, they are now technology-wise and computer-literate. Their profession has moved to improve their academic status with professors, researchers, senior lecturers and the like, who are able to respond and comment on all aspects of health care. They can now tell me the causes and management of acute respiratory, cardiac, renal, hepatic or multi-organ failure.

Nevertheless, I have wondered.

With all this new-found knowledge comes a sense of empowerment. If their new talents are unable to be put into practice, frustration and anger will surface. They have an opinion about all aspects concerning the standard of care for the critically ill patient. And why shouldn't they? Perhaps they had an opinion previously but kept it to themselves. Treatment concerning the circulation, ventilation, sedation, plasma biochemistry, urinary output and even systemic vascular resistance (SVR) will be questioned. For example: "Mrs. Smith's SVR is 2000 - are you happy about that?"

I once use to attempt to give a short discourse on circulatory physiology to explain why I was not necessarily 'happy about that' but under the set of circumstances that the patient was encountering I would tolerate it - to find a few hours later that a nursing note would be added to state that Dr. Worthley was notified and was 'happy about that.' I have also been informed after I had prescribed vecuronium for a 'posturing' patient, that "I'm not happy about giving this patient a relaxant unless he is also given some sedation" even though the patient was deeply unconscious with a large intracerebral haemorrhage.

Intensive care patients and their problems are complex. Normal physiological values that include a mean arterial pressure of 80 mmHg, PaO_2 of 90 mmHg and urine output of 50 mL/hr are sometimes not normal for various pathological conditions. A PaO_2 of 60 mmHg, urine output of 10 mL/hr, and arterial pressure of 60 mmHg or 120 mmHg may be acceptable as an alternative to large doses of vasoactive agents, intubation and ventilation or extensive use of diuretics. Furthermore, sedation and opiates may be inappropriate for those who are in a coma. To simply change a number that we measure, or add an agent to suppress consciousness that is already suppressed, is not necessarily associated with improved patient outcome.

Moreover, while intensive care nurses have become more informed, I often wondered if this aspect of their training has received more attention than the various practical aspects of their vocation, such as securing endotracheal tubes, underwater seal drains or central venous lines (which occasionally appear to just 'fall out'), zeroing pressure transducers, checking the endotracheal cuff, ensuring vasoactive infusions are administered in separate lines, the nasogastric suction is working, administering intravenous antibiotics without delay, managing pressure areas and attending to eye and mouth hygiene.

Nonetheless, any sense of medical paternalism or arrogance is no longer accepted by nurses, physiotherapists, junior medical staff or hospital cleaners. Nor should it have been. All wish to be an active partner in the decision-making process relating to the patient's management. However, and more so now, if these expectations are unfulfilled, the nurse, junior medical staff or physiotherapist (or hospital cleaner) is likely to consult their supervisor, administrator, lawyer or local newspaper reporter, as they are no longer frightened of confrontation. To be fair though, all believe that they act with the understanding that whatever they do will be in the patient's best interest. Nevertheless, having a committee that decrees treatment often produces the same result as having a committee drive a car.

Inside God's Shed

Rather than having one coordinated team, two or more teams exist with all hands tugging at the wheel to produce the erratic results that nobody takes responsibility for.

I guess as a 'baby boomer' wishing to judge the change in those who are largely 'generation X' I risk being pilloried as just another dinosaur who has outlived his hope and who should be relegated to the retirement 'condo'. Yet to live through the gestation of the discipline I know as intensive care medicine and see its maturation may allow one a useful perspective.

With all these random thoughts circling about concerning the change in the relationship between the intensive care specialist and nurse, I felt somewhat repentant following a recent incident. A patient was admitted to our intensive care unit following coronary artery bypass surgery. In this group of patients we often use intravenous sodium nitroprusside (SNP) to keep the mean arterial pressure ranging between 60 to 90 mmHg. In one such patient I found the mean arterial pressure had increased to 100 mmHg and asked the nurse "how is Mr. Jones?"

"OK," she replied "the pressure is up a bit so I have turned the SNP off." I looked at the pump and, sure enough, it was off. I leaned over, reset it and turned it on again. Just then Jan (the intensive care charge nurse) appeared.

"I think nurse might have a few questions to ask you, Jan," I said and left.

The next day I received a letter from the nurse that said: "Thank you for your patience yesterday. I was so nervous and anxious about making sure that I was organised and did everything correctly, that I ended up making stupid errors. Unfortunately anxiety gains its own momentum which does not dissipate easily. I will never repeat that error again and will keep trying to deliver the best patient care I can."

Intensive care units are stressful places and I guess I tend to forget how stressful they are to junior staff. I reflected a little and felt that perhaps when making judgements about the various changes in intensive care I should remember my early days better.

Lately, I think I have listened a little more.

The power of magic

"Do not try to live forever. You will not succeed."
George Bernard Shaw

Patients are vulnerable. No more so than those who have an incurable disease. When the time comes to give a prognosis, while they may appear to accept the sentence, most likely he or she denies the verdict and it is only when constant pain or distress occur that the reality of the disease becomes apparent. Alternative forms of medicine flourish in such an environment, promising everything, but often, and cruelly, delivering nothing.

Recently, a patient was admitted to our intensive care unit for the fourth time with an episode of acute-on-chronic respiratory failure. She was in her 70's and during the last five years required home oxygen for chronic hypoxia caused by a progressive and restrictive kyphoscoliosis with severe right heart failure. She had been, at best, wheelchair bound, although during the last 6 months she rarely ventured from her bedroom and was managed with the continuous help of her doting husband and three daughters. Her respiratory physician had advised the family 5 years ago that she would not live for more than two years. On the morning of her admission she was found unconscious in bed and was transported rapidly to hospital for further management.

After I had intubated and settled the patient on a ventilator, I told her daughters that their mother would once again require 'life support' but that this time it would probably be for a prolonged period, if not for the remainder of her life, as there seemed to be no acute reversible factor. To my surprise, their first request was:

"Could mum have her antioxidant and inhalation treatment continued please?"

"What are they?" I asked, readying myself for anything.

It appeared that three weeks ago, on the advice of a friend, a naturopath had been called who prescribed a 6-hourly inhalation of a colloidal silver solution and a weekly intravenous infusion of a solution containing 20 g vitamin C, 5 g of magnesium sulphate, 5 mg pyridoxine and homeopathic amounts of zinc and copper. The intravenous medication was supplied and administered by the naturopath who also advised discontinuation of her regular medications and against future hospital visits. He told them that the antioxidant and inhaled silver 'treatment' had worked miracles in many of his patients for a diverse range of disorders that had been declared incurable by the medical profession.

After meeting the congenial therapist, they embarked upon his recommendations and it was not long before they were convinced that their mother was being kept alive by his treatment.

"But you've come to hospital in spite of the naturopath's advice?" I said, hoping to find some reason for their return to conventional medicine while still remaining fixed to their naturopathic alternative.

"Oh, we want all the help that we can get," was the reply, confirming the desperate and inconsistent approach taken by patients and relatives of terminally ill patients.

"Yet your mother has deteriorated with the antioxidant and inhaled therapy?" I said still trying to find logic.

"They haven't had time to fully work yet," they said eagerly, and repeated the unanswerable question that often haunts every practitioner managing patients with an incurable disease "and what have we got to lose?"

I desperately wanted to say "but it's been more than three weeks. . . ." and "where is the evidence . . . ?", but didn't, as I felt that this would stretch the point and I wasn't about to change their position.

In general, the public are neither familiar nor convinced by the scientific process. The benefits or otherwise of homeopathy, herbalism and hypnosis for various 'incurable' disorders are usually confirmed by testimonials and anecdotal reports. It seems that if it cannot be understood, the mechanism is validated. The magical and mysterious go hand in hand. The fact that a friend did not respond to being immersed in warm goat's milk has far more meaning than the fact that the process makes no sense. Yet negative anecdotes are rarely, if ever, told (often to save embarrassment), a fact that only adds weight to those stories, which are readily told, where orthodox medicine 'failed' and a miracle occurred.

Nonetheless, orthodox medicine has its own problems.[1] Even proponents of evidence-based medicine can be emotionally tied to their beliefs.[2] While it is easy to criticise an eccentric practice and hold the medically accepted aloof, in an individual case, a practice that poses little harm may sometimes be better tolerated than ridiculed.

"What happened to your patient?" you ask.

The infused antioxidants and inhaled silver were discontinued as the relatives were amenable to some reasoning. For example, we measured the plasma ascorbic acid, magnesium, zinc and copper levels and found them to be either extremely high or at least above the upper limit of normal. We also cultured a light growth of *Pseudomonas aeruginosa* from the sputum, which became a heavy growth after 24 hr of the nebulised colloidal silver. Nevertheless, the family provided a quartz crystal which they believed would act as a substitute for the antioxidants and inhaled silver. We kept this under her pillow. The patient remained mechanically ventilated for two months and after a prolonged period of weaning, and ignoring blood gas and pulse oximetry measurements, was finally transferred home. She died one day later.

REFERENCES
1. Worthley LIG. Can a doctor enjoy a medical company's generosity without prescribing its products? Crit Care Resus 2002;4:323-324.
2. Chalmers I. Human albumin administration in critically ill patients. I would not want an albumin transfusion. BMJ 1998;317:885.

Conventional medicine, complementary medicine and alternative medicine, or should they just be called medicine and unproven beliefs?

"There are, in fact, two things, science and opinion; the former begets knowledge, the latter ignorance."
Hippocrates

"G'day Rob. Long time no see!" I said.
"Yep, it's been a while."
So began the conversation, via Skype, with a friend I had not seen for about 40 years. He left Australia for New York then moved to San Francisco to run his own software company, which he later sold. He then became interested, among other things, in the power of the mind to heal.
"Still doing medicine?" he asked.
"For a few more years," I replied.
"I might just send you something."
Following our call he emailed me a video by Bruce Lipton, a PhD researcher who had published a book, 'The Biology of Belief: Unleashing the Power of Consciousness, Matter and Miracles.' The video lasted for 30 minutes and discussed the potential power of the mind to help an individual recover from any illness, as messages emanating from our positive and negative thoughts could control our DNA. I sent a reasonably measured response back to Rob stating, in brief, that while the mind has a powerful influence in certain disorders (e.g. a placebo effect), for it to cure terminal illnesses and to stop ageing, I felt, drew a fairly long bow.
At about the same time, another friend called me and asked about 714-X for treating cancer of the stomach. It transpired that his daughter-in-law had undergone a total gastrectomy for stomach cancer

and, as there had been a secondary spread of the cancer, she decided to embark upon alternative therapy with 714-X. Trawling the web, I found that the proponents of 714-X therapy claim that a disease can be diagnosed and monitored by noting the number and forms of tiny living particles in the blood called somatids, and that 714-X therapy cures cancer by interfering with the movement of somatids throughout the bloodstream.[1] After accessing all the standard scientific literature, I replied that there was no evidence for the existence of somatids, or any beneficial effect of 714-X in the treatment of cancer. It was an unproven treatment based on an unfounded mechanism.

In an intensive care medical practice, complementary and alternative medical (CAM) therapies are rare, but not unknown.[2] However, as we often deal with terminal illness I began thinking about the influence of CAM therapies in conventional medical management. Surveys have shown that up to 50% of the population use CAM in one form or another,[3,4,5] with a current annual global expenditure of these therapies approximating $50 billion.[5] The question is why do intelligent and perceptive people believe in alternative medicine? Is it because they feel conventional medicine does not have all the answers and desperation leads them to illogical thinking;[6] or perhaps a 'what have we got to lose' argument motivates them when conventional medicine advises a poor prognosis? We all want therapy that works. Do we simply differ in what we believe is evidence?

Conventional medicine uses randomised controlled clinical trials (RCT's) to investigate both safety and efficacy of a test treatment compared with a control,[7] and considers any new treatment doubtful until proven otherwise. The results of RCT's are reviewed by experts to ensure that they meet certain standards before being accepted and published (i.e. peer-reviewed). Treatments that are tested in this way are called 'evidence-based'. Complementary and alternative medicine, on the other hand, use testimonials and anecdotes as evidence of efficacy, and believe that a new treatment is valid until unproven.[8,9]

However, the statement 'that there is no alternative medicine. There is only scientifically proven, evidence-based medicine, supported by solid data, or unproven medicine, for which scientific evidence is lacking'[10,11] can overlook the benefit that some patients derive from

CAM therapies. For instance, they enhance quality of life, improve well-being and control symptoms such as pain, stress, fatigue, depression and anxiety. In this regard, the Cancer Council of Australia[12] and the American Cancer Society[13] separate complementary therapy from alternative therapy.

They view complementary therapy as that which includes counseling, peer support groups, relaxation, meditation, hypnosis, music and physical therapies (e.g. massage, yoga, tai chi, Pilates). These techniques do not cure cancer; they supplement conventional medical treatment and can be useful by enhancing the patient's quality of life. Alternative therapy, on the other hand, includes bizarre diets, naturopathy, immune therapy, biofeedback, reflexology, crystals, homeopathy, chelation, detox, herbs and megavitamins. They are not scientifically proven, can be harmful, are often used instead of conventional medicine and are usually promoted as 'cures' using terms such as 'energy fields', 'aura', 'resonance' and 'channelling'. They may be identified by the claim that they, can cure all cancers, are something that can only be administered by certain people, have no side effects and are justifiably expensive.

While some promote alternative medicine for financial gain there are others who genuinely believe that their therapy works,[8] and confusion often exists when the patient receives alternative therapy and gets better – surely it has been due to the treatment?

However this assumes that the diagnosis is correct. It also uses the *post hoc ergo propter hoc* (Latin: after this, therefore, because of this) reasoning error that ignores the natural history of the disease, regression to the mean and the placebo effect. For example, a common cold will resolve within 7 days irrespective of treatment and a patient will always seek help when they are at their sickest with symptoms waning later in spite of treatment (i.e. regression to the mean).[14] The *placebo* (Latin: I will please) effect describes any treatment that is beneficial only if administered to a patient who is aware that he or she is receiving the treatment. The critical component of the placebo is an expectation of benefit by the patient, and has been long recognised as the pharmacologically and physiologically inactive component of treatment.[15] However, its effect usually lasts for a short time only, and has little if any clinically important benefit except in the treatment of pain, nausea, depression and anxiety.[16,17] Acupuncture, in particular, has been the subject of many randomised, controlled clinical studies to treat a variety disorders, all of which have shown that there is no scientific evidence to support the benefits beyond a placebo effect.[5,14,15]

If there is a negative patient expectation, the agent may cause unpleasant or worsening symptoms (e.g. headaches, nervousness, nausea, or constipation), a response known as the *nocebo* (Latin: I will harm) effect. One randomized controlled study of 1800 postoperative cardiac bypass patients found a nocebo effect in patients who were told that they would receive intercessory prayer postoperatively.[18] Another report, however, summarising 10 prospective randomized clinical trials concerning intercessory prayer concluded "the evidence does not support a recommendation either in favour or against the use of intercessory prayer."[19]

One of the most widely used CAM treatments is dietary supplements, which include vitamins, minerals, herbs, animal parts, algae, yeasts, fungus, and many other food substances or extracts (e.g. powdered amino acids, enzymes, energy bars, and liquid food supplements). Vitamins, in particular, are marketed with celebrity endorsements of: "works for me", "I can't get by without it", "it brightens my day" or "gives me more energy". They don't claim to cure a disease and often state that they improve vitality, energy and concentration. Nevertheless, no matter what the claim is, apart from a documented vitamin deficiency, periconceptional folic acid supplements in women to reduce the risk of neural tube defects,[20] and a placebo effect, vitamin supplements are not therapeutic.

While there may be an occasional worthwhile remedy in the thousands of herbs currently marketed, scientific reviews by the Cochrane Collaboration have found only 6 agents to date to be more effective than placebo. Even these reviews usually add several caveats to their conclusions suggesting that more rigorous RCT's are required to confirm their efficacy, and their long-term effects are unknown. The six agents are: *St John's wort* which may be more effective than placebo in treating major depression[21] (although it can alter the metabolism of warfarin, cyclosporine, digoxin, amitryptilline, theophylline, tacrolimus, paroxitine and should not be used with these agents),[22] both *Devil's Claw* (Harpagophytum Procumbens) and *White Willow Bark* (Salix Alba) may reduce low back pain more than placebo,[23] *Hawthorn* (Crataegus spp.) is a vasodilator and may be more effective than placebo in improving chronic heart failure symptoms,[24] *Horse chestnut* (Aesculus hippocastanum) seed extract reduced leg pain, oedema and pruritus when compared with placebo in patients with chronic venous insufficiency,[25] and *Kava extract* (Piper methylsticum) may be superior compared with placebo as a treatment for anxiety.[26]

I remember as a medical student watching the consultation between a senior rheumatologist, who had an unfortunate stutter, and one of his patients. It was *circa* 1967 and at a time when aspirin was the predominant therapy for any rheumatic condition. The patient was an elderly woman. When the time for her outpatient review finally arrived he helped her through the door and steered her to the consultation room chair. The rheumatologist remained by her side and said his usual introductory:

"Well how are you M-M-M-Mrs. Smith?"

"Oh, doctor, I am so much better. I have used a copper wrist bracelet for the last 4 weeks and it has helped my arthritis enormously," she gushed.

"That's m-m-m-marvellous," he replied. "It's not an inconvenience?" he asked.

"No" she replied.

"Are you s-s-s-still taking your Palaprin Forte?" (an aluminium acetylsalicylate product that is now no longer available in Australia), he enquired.

"Well, I've reduced the dose to alternate days and I think that it makes me feel better," she said, looking at both her hands.

"Well, we will continue with that regimen and we'll see if your p-p-p-pain remains at bay."

She gave him a big smile and with that he helped her onto the examination couch, examined the upper and lower limb movements and after a few other formalities we ushered her outside, with a blood form for a serum salycilate estimation and a note to arrange for another outpatient appointment in one month's time.

As we returned to his room I said, "You didn't tell her that there is no scientific evidence of any benefit using copper bangles?"

"Well n-n-no," he said as he returned to his desk to write down his findings, "You see if I tried to em-em-em.... embarrass her with an im-im-im-impolite remark about a harmless thing such as a copper bangle. What would have that achieved?"

"Exactly!" I thought.

REFERENCES
1. American Cancer Society. http://www.cancer.org/Treatment/ TreatmentsandSideEffects/ComplementaryandAlternativeMedicine/PharmacologicalandBiologicalTreatment/714-x. (accessed April 2012)
2. Worthley LIG. The power of magic. Crit Care Resusc 2003;5:69-70.
3. Eisenberg DM, Davis RB, Ettner SL, Appel S, Wilkey S, Van Rompay M, et al.Trends in alternative medicine use in the United States, 1990-1997: results of a follow-up national survey. JAMA 1998;280:1569-1575.
4. Tindle HA, Davis RB, Phillips RS, Eisenberg DM. Trends in use of complementary and alternative medicine by US adults: 1997-2002. Altern Ther Health Med. 2005;11:42-49.
5. Sing S, Ernst E. Trick or treatment? Alternative medicine on trial. London: Bantam Press, 2008.
6. Holland JC. Use of alternative medicine – a marker for distress? N Engl J Med 1999;340:1758-1759.
7. US Food and Drug Administration. http://www.fda.gov/.(accessed April 2012).
8. Fitzgerald FT. Science and scam: Alternative thought patterns in alternative health care. N Engl J Med 1984;309:1066-1067.
9. Fitzgerald FT. Alternative health care. N Engl J Med 1984;310:791-792.
10. Fontanarosa PB, Lundberg GD. Alternative medicine meets science. JAMA 1998;280:1618-1619.

11. Alternative medicine- the risks of untested and unregulated remedies. Angell M, Kassirer JP. N Engl J Med 1998;339:839-841.
12. Cancer Council of Australia. http://www.cancer.org.au//aboutcancer/ complementaryandalternativetherapies.htm. (accessed March 2012)
13. American Cancer Society. http://www.cancer.org/Treatment/ TreatmentsandSideEffects/ComplementaryandAlternativeMedicin e/complementary-and-alternative-methods-for-cancer-management. (accessed March 2012)
14. Thompson WG. The placebo effect and health: combining science and compassionate care. New York: Prometheus Books, 2005.
15. Barker Bausell R. Snake oil science: the truth about complementary and alternative medicine. New York: Oxford University Press, 2007
16. Hróbjartsson A, Gøtzsche PC. Is the placebo powerless? An analysis of clinical trials comparing placebo with no treatment. N Engl J Med 2001;344:1594-1602.
17. Hróbjartsson A, Gøtzsche PC (20 January 2010). Placebo interventions for all clinical conditions. Cochrane Database Syst Rev 2010;106: CD003974
18. Benson H, Dusek JA, Sherwood JB, Lam P, Bethea CF, Carpenter W, et al. Study of the Therapeutic Effects of Intercessory Prayer (STEP) in cardiac bypass patients: a multicenter randomized trial of uncertainty and certainty of receiving intercessory prayer. Am Heart J 2006;151:934-942.
19. Roberts L, Ahmed I, Hall S, Davison A. Intercessory prayer for the alleviation of ill health. Cochrane Database Syst Rev 2009 Apr 15;(2):CD000368.
20. De-Rigil LM, Fernández-Gaxiola AC, Dowswell T, Peña-Rosas JP. Effects and safety of periconceptional folate supplementation for preventing birth defects. Cochrane Database Syst Rev 2010 Oct 6;(10):CD007950.
21. Linde K, Berner MM, Kriston L. St John's wort for major depression. Cochrane Database Syst Rev 2008 Oct 8;(4): CD000448.

22. De Smet PAGM. Herbal remedies. N Engl J Med 2002;347:2046-2056.
23. Gagnier JJ, van Tulder M, Berman B, Bombardier C. Herbal medicine for low back pain. Cochrane Database Syst Rev 2006 Apr 19;(2):CD004504.
24. Pittler MH, Guo R, Ernst E. Hawthorn extract for treating chronic heart failure. Cochrane Database Syst Rev 2008 Jan 23;(1): CD005312.
25. Pittler MH, Ernst E. Horse chestnut seed extract for chronic venous insufficiency. Cochrane Database Syst Rev 2006 Jan 25;(1):CD003230.
26. Pittler MH, Ernst E. Kava extract for treating anxiety. Cochrane Database Syst Rev 2002;(2):CD003383.

Bedside peer review: standards, judgement and sweet charity

"Judge not, that ye be not judged. For with what judgment ye judge, ye shall be judged: and with what measure ye mete, it shall be measured to you."
Matthew 7:1-2

Intensive care medicine is like no other specialty, in that we work in very close quarters with our peers. We hand over patients at the end of our shift and take over from others at the end of their shift. Within such an arrangement we have a unique view of our colleague's work and often judge, either overtly or covertly, the standard of care we perceive they practice. Working in such close proximity may even provoke one or more of the seven deadly sins (e.g. envy, pride, wrath). Fragile egos can get bruised when the care of a patient is handed over to another, treatment is altered and the patient gets better. Worse still, a diagnosis is made that has been missed by the predecessor.

Early in my career, I worked in an intensive care unit where the approach by one of my peers to the critically ill patient, I felt, was of a more 'considered' ('ponderous' or 'slow' are probably not the right words) nature than mine. As the fellow also had an anaesthetic list on one day in his working week, I often wondered if he 'weaned' his patients from the ventilator at the end of each surgical procedure. Nevertheless, during his week 'on', while patients may have been extubated later than would have occurred during my rostered week, they always seemed to survive while under his care. In retrospect, they may have even prospered. Moreover, this gentle practitioner taught me the power of tenacity in the management of an intensive care patient. He believed that if a critically ill patient "lasts for a week; they shouldn't die", a lesson I found valuable in 'pressing on' during the management of patients who appear not to improve with therapy, but refuse to die, and in trying to understand the edge of possibility and the beginning of futility.

105

That there are differences in the practice of intensive care clinicians is not in doubt. The nurses and trainee medical staff often state provocatively "but Dr. X doesn't do that - he does Y." I tend to explain that I cannot comment on his or her practice, but can only explain my own practice, stating that in a teaching institution the strength of a unit is in the *reasoned* disparity of practice. With an exposure to as many different approaches to the management of a patient, an environment is created where sound medical judgement can be learnt, as the predicted and real outcomes can be carefully observed by the trainee.

Even with evidence-based medicine, clinical practice often presents cases that do not 'fit' the inclusion criteria of a 'landmark' study. Judgement is difficult in such cases and treatment will inevitably vary between practitioners. One study even found that the same practitioner, given the same clinical problem, often varied his or her advice with time.[1]

It is almost impossible to judge a peer's practice without exhibiting positive or negative bias, particularly when judging one who works within the same institution. If we are asked to do so informally, our opinion is probably best kept to ourselves, particularly if it is a disparaging one. However, if we are asked to give a formal opinion concerning a colleague's practice, then while our judgment must be sound and cogent, particularly within a legal environment, it must be tempered with humility and understanding.

To assess the standard of medical care and the 'culture of care' within a given intensive care unit, a regular unit audit is often performed. This may take the form of a review of a patient's management irrespective of the outcome (e.g. a monthly random selection of case records to review whether the care was acceptable, or whether a change in the care would have altered the patient's outcome), or a review of morbidity and mortality during a defined period (e.g. a monthly death audit, or review of specific medical complications).[2] The review of the medical care of a patient who survives is easily tempered with humility and understanding, as a sound medical practice is inferred with the patient's survival. On the other hand, reviewing the care of a patient who died, poor medical management is often implied even though death may be the result of good medical practice just as much as bad medical practice. What is easily forgotten, is that death is the end point of life well managed, as well as an adverse outcome of a therapeutic intervention.

Nevertheless, a death review may be useful in considering the unit's overall standard of care. Particularly when reviewing issues such as 'futility' where a reflex response to critical illness by considering the most pessimistic outcome may result in the patient receiving less than optimal care, contributing to a self-fulfilling prophecy.[3] This approach can easily breed an acceptance of substandard practice and a culture where withdrawal of therapy becomes commonplace. On the other hand, admission of patients with terminal conditions is also wrong, as it wastes an expensive resource and reduces staff morale.

However, audits are not flawless. Even a death review audit may not detect an aberrant practice. Part of a report of an audit of the practice of the former family doctor Harold Shipman carried out in January 1998, stated, "Great to see a single-handed enthusiastic GP with a rolling programme of audit – keep up the good work."[4] This report occurred just 9 months before the arrest that led to his conviction for killing 15 patients. An official enquiry concluded that he was probably responsible for at least 200 more murders.

As with any judgement, there are no short cuts. The process has to be impartial. An audit of any clinical practice requires one who has the necessary experience, vigilance and charity to provide a report that is credible and just.

REFERENCES
1. Rutkow IM. Surgical decision making. The reproducibility of clinical judgement. Arch Surg 1982;117:337-340.
2. Brook RH, McGlynn EA, Cleary PD. Quality of health care. Part 2: measuring quality of care. N Engl J Med 1996;335:966-970.
3. Siegler M. Pascal's wager and the hanging of crepe. N Engl J Med 1975;293:853-857.
4. Fitzpatrick M. Auditing deaths. Lancet 2003;362(9383):586.

"Do you wish your husband to be resuscitated?"

"There is no judgment more dangerous than that someone else's life is not worth living. The passing of this judgment can all too easily become habit."
Theodore Dalrymple

Asking a wife to sign a 'not-for-resuscitation' (NFR) order, before explaining exactly what was happening to her husband, disturbed me somewhat. Yes, the patient was ill, he had myelodysplasia with bilateral subdural haematomas and staphylococcal septicaemia, and, yes, these were serious problems, but her husband 'Bill' was well a few weeks ago and needed only an occasional transfusion to manage his anaemia. Why did she need to sign a 'not-for-resuscitation' order? Hadn't he always wanted to be treated actively?

I was phoned by his wife – a long-term friend of both my wife and I – saying, "I have just been given a form by my local doctor, asking me to consider whether I should sign a not-for-resuscitation order for Bill. Is this what I should do?"

"What?" I exclaimed incredulously.

Bill had a 12 month history of myelodysplasia. Three months ago he developed atrial fibrillation and was anticoagulated to prepare him for cardioversion. During the three-week period of anticoagulation which followed his cardioversion, he developed two small subdural haematomas. After being reviewed by a neurosurgeon, it was decided that conservative management (e.g. vitamin K and platelet transfusions) with close observation would be the right course. He was sent back to his rural community to be managed by his local doctor and have sporadic transfusions for his anaemia at the district hospital. However, the intravascular catheter used for his most recent transfusion became infected, leading to a *Staphylococcus aureus* septicaemia.

Inside God's Shed

He remained at the district hospital, hypotensive, pyrexial and confused and was obviously thought by the local doctor to be dying.

"Helen," I said, "ignore the form and tell the doctor to immediately call an ambulance to transport him to the Flinders Medical Centre intensive care unit. I will notify whoever is on duty there to expect him and that he is for full resuscitation."

I don't know why I felt so troubled. Perhaps it is because if things get too hard for some clinicians, they would prefer to opt for the easy life. Get the patient to sign the NFR form, turn the morphine on and we can all go home. It is difficult to hide your feelings of outrage from the relatives, who need to be assured that everything is going to plan and that the local doctor is doing his best. I dearly wanted to say to Helen, "call your local doctor and say 'send Bill to the Flinders Medical Centre because they will have someone there who will *really* care'" but that would help no one. The family would forever loose trust with their local doctor, who may be the only clinician in the district, who is overworked, underappreciated and does not need his reputation to be tarnished by a smart-aleck ICU specialist.

Bill subsequently had a long and complicated illness. His septicaemia required 6 weeks of intravenous flucloxacillin, he underwent bilateral craniotomies to remove the subdural haematomas, and finally had a partial bone marrow transplant as his myelodysplasia had rapidly worsened requiring daily platelet transfusions, weekly blood transfusions, and an occasional white cell transfusion to maintain his neutrophil count above critical levels.

Four months later he was home, taking a 'grocery list' of drugs including atenolol, fexofenadine, esomeprazole, magnesium aspartate, famciclovir, posaconazole suspension, sulphamethoxazole and trimethopim, cyclosporin, symbicort and spiriva. He had a bald head (his eyebrows were growing again), needed an afternoon nap, but had the old glint back in his eye. He reckons that the medical and nursing teams who treated him in both hospitals were marvellous and he still has faith in his local doctor who has been amazed at his progress and probably regrets reaching so hastily for the NFR form.

Quality control, risk and adverse events in the intensive care unit

"there were incidents and accidents, there were hints and allegations."
Paul Simon

The assessment of the quality of medical practice in a hospital is often determined by a medical audit. Another way of assessing standard of care is by prospectively collecting morbidity and mortality data. One such method is by incident monitoring where incidents, or adverse events, are defined as events or circumstances that could have, or did, harm a patient following any medical encounter.[1]

An 'adverse event' occurrence rate of 2% - 4% in a general medical population is often quoted,[2,3] although some believe that it is closer to 50%.[4] In the USA, more people die in a given year as a result of medical errors than from motor vehicle accidents, breast cancer or AIDS.[5,6]

In an Australian review of medical records for more than 14000 admissions to 28 hospitals, an adverse event, which resulted in disability or a longer hospital stay for the patient, was noted in 16.6% of admissions. Fifty one percent of the adverse events were considered preventable, and in 4.9% the patient died.[7] However, this study was subject to much criticism. For example, it was not a prospective study and was not subjected to critical review before release, raising the question of bias.[8] Moreover, 45% of deaths occurred after patients were admitted for life-saving therapy (i.e. were at risk of imminent death regardless of treatment) and the study did not attempt to measure the benefits of the health care provided (i.e. it was not a risk/benefit study). Nevertheless, it did highlight the fact that 'adverse events' do occur in Australian hospitals, and while hospital care has become safer over the last 20 years,[9] there is still a need for improvement.

Inside God's Shed

There is evidence, as one might expect, that adverse events are not well tolerated in the critically ill patient, with the consequences of any error likely to be more significant.[3,10] In an Australian study of critically ill patients from seven intensive care units, 610 critical incidents were reported.[11] Children appear to be at particular risk.[12,13] In one study the error rate was greater in the paediatric intensive care unit (PICU) compared with the normal ward or neonatal intensive care unit, due to the greater heterogeneity of patients cared for in the PICU and the broad range of drugs and dosages used.[14] Medication-related errors also increase as the average number of drugs administered increases, explaining the higher incidence of medication-related errors in critically ill patients when compared with standard ward patients.[15]

While the method of incident monitoring has been used successfully in improving the aerospace and nuclear energy industries,[16] in the ICU it can be a blunt instrument when used to assess and improve the quality of medical care. For instance, recording of events are often at variance with what had actually happened.[17] Furthermore, I could conceive that almost any happening in the ICU would constitute an event or circumstance that could have or would have harmed the patient. In any ICU, whether on home or foreign soil, at least one 'incident' can be revealed per ward round, if not per patient, to the experienced eye - if one had a mind to just sit and watch all the activity that involved the patient during a 24 hour period. These deficiencies often persist even after attempts have been made to help the staff comply with the required standard. To give just two examples: poor compliance with the requirement for hand washing by medical and nursing staff between patient examinations and procedures in the ICU,[18,19,20,21,22,23,24,25,26] and incorrect zero referencing for haemodynamic measurements.[27] Both are notorious and persistent ICU 'incidents' and one could speculate quite reasonably that harm could have occurred or did occur to the patient with either.

However, before we add the sign 'All hope abandon, ye who enter here' to the front door of the ICU, it is probably better to do a regular review of patient morbidity and mortality to determine the type of adverse events (Table 1)[28] and attempt to prioritise the severity of these events. One should then review the cause, frequency and outcome of the severe events rather than detailing the minor transgressions.

Table 1. Type of adverse events

Diagnostic
    Error or delay in diagnosis
    Failure to employ tests that were indicated
    Failure to see results of tests
    Failure to act on results of monitoring or testing

Treatment
    Error in the performance of an operation, procedure or test
    Error in administering the treatment
    Error in the dose or method of using a drug
    Avoidable delay in treatment or in responding to an abnormal test
    Inappropriate (i.e. not indicated) care

Preventive
    Failure to provide prophylactic treatment
    Inadequate monitoring or follow-up of treatment

Other
    Failure of communication
    Equipment failure
    Other system failure

Adverse events are either preventable (e.g. administering penicillin to a patient with a known penicillin allergy) or unpreventable (e.g. a patient with pneumococcal pneumonia with no history of a penicillin allergy who has an allergic reaction to penicillin). However if they are the result of a 'calculated' risk (e.g. an elderly patient with an acute myocardial infarction who is treated with a thrombolytic agent who develops a cerebral haemorrhage) it often becomes a matter of opinion rather than fact as to how they should be classified.[29]

In general, the community expects clinicians to function without error, as errors are usually perceived to be due to carelessness or incompetence and therefore due to negligence.[30] This means that the clinician is expected to be infallible - which is impossible. In the instance of a 'calculated' risk, the community tends to accept a greater risk when it is voluntary than when it is imposed, hence informed consent for any procedure is important. The aim is to judge fairly whether the 'calculated' risk was warranted when reviewing any adverse outcome.

Preventable adverse events that do not result in harm represent an opportunity to improve care.[31,32] Those that do result in harm also represent litigious opportunities, and usually discourage accurate reporting of errors, with attempts often being made to shift the emphasis from preventable to unpreventable or, at least, to an acceptable 'calculated' risk. While clinicians must be vigilant and held accountable for their actions, sheeting home blame for past errors rather than understanding their cause will not improve quality and standard of health care. Negligence is a matter for the courts. Quality of care is a matter for the medical profession.

Quality of care incorporates three aspects:
1. Customisation (i.e. to inform the patient, or relative, of the options, complications and likely outcome of all alternatives)
2. Provision of services in a manner that is consistent with current medical knowledge and best practices (there is often a great deal of variability in this)
3. Provision of services free from accidental injury.

Some believe that the development of policies, procedures and protocols will improve care. Protocols assume that if rigidly defined paths are followed, the correct diagnosis and treatment will be achieved.[33] The assumption arises from the belief that every experiment performed under the same conditions produces the same result. However, there are important limitations to a blind application of this principle, as the pathophysiology of disease is often poorly understood and patients vary in their reaction to an illness and response to treatment. Furthermore, patients and physicians may vary in what they believe is the best outcome. For example, while beta-blockers may reduce the mortality in acute myocardial infarction, the patient may not be willing to take the drug due to a reduced sense of well-being. To some, the smallest fragment of life is valuable, whereas to others any restriction to comfort and activity is intolerable. While some protocols have been successful (e.g. weaning from the ventilator) in general they do not supplant sound clinical judgement.[34]

Unlike protocols and policies, guidelines are a little softer and are defined as 'systematically developed statements to assist practitioner and patient decisions about appropriate health care for specific clinical circumstances'[35] using evidence-based medicine. Nevertheless, many studies have failed to detect any lasting impact of clinical practice guidelines on clinical practice or patient outcomes.[36] Moreover, guidelines are not infrequently biased, with one report finding 59% of the experts who participated in the formulation of clinical practice guidelines had financial relationships with companies whose drugs were considered in the guidelines they authored.[37]

The way to improve quality is to focus on the collection of data that will allow the development of appropriate remediation systems to prevent future errors.[10] One should try to understand the underlying cause, so that factors responsible (e.g. poor knowledge or judgement, fatigue or excessive stress, reliance upon memory, inexperience) can be changed.[30] Also of importance is an active intensive care medicine training, education and research program as this provides the environment necessary to develop a culture that changes an unsound practices.

Returning to the notorious and persistent ICU hand washing and zero referencing incidents, in any human activity there are times when everything cannot be perfect. Concerning hand washing, while I believe that it should be performed between patient examinations and procedures, it may be better to 'scrupulously' enforce it when it really matters (e.g. in isolating patients who have methicillin resistant *Staphylococcus aureus*, as hand washing has been shown to significantly reduce its spread)[38] rather than attempt to enforce it for all patients. Arthur Rudolph (a scientist who developed the Saturn 5 rocket that launched the first Apollo mission to the moon) stated this principle as: 'you want a valve that doesn't leak and you try everything possible to

Inside God's Shed

develop one. But the real world provides you with a leaky valve. You have to determine how much leaking you can tolerate.'

REFERENCES
1. Wright D, Mackenzie SJ, Buchan I, Cairns CS, Price LE. Critical incidents in the intensive therapy unit. Lancet 1991;338(8768):676-678.
2. Thomas EJ, Studdert DM, Newhouse JP, Zbar BI, Howard KM, Williams EJ, et al. Costs of medical injuries in Utah and Colorado. Inquiry 1999;36:255-264.
3. Brennan TA, Leape LL, Laird NM, Hebert L, Localio AR, Lawthers AG, et al. Incidence of adverse events and negligence in hospitalised patients: Results of the Harvard Medical Practice Study I. N Engl J Med 1991; 324:370-376.
4. Krizek TJ. Medical errors: reporting and punishment. Lancet 2000;356(9231):773.
5. Centers for Disease Control and Prevention (National Centre for Health Statistics). Births and Deaths: Preliminary Data for 1998. National Vital Statistics Reports. 1999;47(25):6.
6. Centers for Disease Control and Prevention (National Centre for Health Statistics). Deaths: Final Data for 1997. National Vital Statistics Reports. 1999;47(19):27.
7. Wilson RM, Runciman WB, Gibberd RW, Harrison BT, Newby L, Hamilton JD. The Quality in Australian Health Care Study. Med J Aust 1995;163:458-471.
8. Relman AS. The Ingelfinger rule. N Engl J Med 1981;305:824-826.
9. Brennan TA. The Institute of Medicine report on medical errors - Could it do harm? N Engl J Med 2000;342:1123-1125.
10. Fraenkel DJ. Safety and quality in intensive care. Crit Care Resusc 2000;2:220-226.
11. Beckmann U, Baldwin I, Hart GK, Runciman WB. The Australian Incident Monitoring Study in Intensive Care: AIMS-ICU. An analysis of the first year of reporting. Anaesth Intensive Care 1996;24:320-329.
12. Koren G, Haslam RH. Pediatric medication errors: predicting and preventing tenfold disasters. J Clin Pharmacol 1994;34:1043-1045.

13. Perlstein PH, Callison C, White M, Barnes B, Edwards NK. Errors in drug computations during newborn intensive care. Am J Dis Child 1979;33:376-379.
14. Folli HL, Pool RL, Benitz WE, Russo JC. Medication error prevention by clinical pharmacists in two children's hospitals. Pediatrics 1987;79:718-722.
15. Cullen DJ, Sweitzer BJ, Bates DW, Burdick E, Edmondson A, Leape LL. Preventable adverse drug events in hospitalized patients: a comparative study of intensive care and general care units. Crit Care Med 1997;25:1289-1297.
16. Bates DW. Error in medicine: what have we learned? Ann Intern Med 2000;132:763-767.
17. Byrne AJ, Jones JG. Inaccurate reporting of simulated critical anaesthetic incidents. Br J Anaesth 1997;78:637-641.
18. Albert RK, Condie F. Hand-washing patterns in medical intensive-care units. N Engl J Med 1981;304:1465-1466.
19. Tibballs J. Teaching hospital medical staff to handwash. Med J Aust 1996;164:395-398.
20. Pittet D, Mourouga P, Perneger TV. Compliance with handwashing in a teaching hospital. Infection Control Program. Ann Intern Med 1999;130:126-130.
21. Steere AC, Mallison GF. Handwashing practices for the prevention of nosocomial infections. Ann Intern Med 1975;83:683-690.
22. Sproat LJ, Inglis TJ. A multicentre survey of hand hygiene practice in intensive care units. J Hosp Infect 1994;26:137-148.
23. Albert RK, Condie F. Hand-washing patterns in medical intensive-care units. N Engl J Med 1981;304:1465-1466.
24. Larson E. Compliance with isolation technique. Am J Infect Control 1983;11:221-225.
25. Meengs MR, Giles BK, Chisholm CD, Cordell WH, Nelson DR. Hand washing frequency in an emergency department. Ann Emerg Med 1994;23:1307-1312.

26. Thompson BL, Dwyer DM, Ussery XT, Denman S, Vacek P, Schwartz B. Handwashing and glove use in a long-term-care facility. Infect Control Hosp Epidemiol 1997;18:97-103.
27. Drake JJ. Locating the external reference point for central venous pressure determination. Nurs Res 1974;23:475-482.
28. Leape LL, Lawthers AG, Brennan TA, Johnson WG. Preventing medical injury. QRB Qual Rev Bull 1993 May;19:144-149.
29. The National Academy of Sciences. To err is human: building a safer health system. http://www.nap.edu/catalog.php?record_id=9728.(accessed April 2011)
30. Leape LL. Error in medicine. JAMA 1994;272:1851-1857.
31. McIntyre N, Popper K. The critical attitude in medicine: the need for a new ethics. Br Med J 1983;287:1919-1923.
32. Blumenthal D. Making medical errors into 'medical treasures'. JAMA 1994;272:1867-1868.
33. Ingelfinger FJ. Algorithms, anyone? N Engl J Med 1973;288:847-848.
34. Ely EW. Challenges encountered in changing physicians' practice styles: the ventilator weaning experience. Intens Care Med 1998;24:539-541.
35. Institute of medicine. Guidelines for clinical practice: from development to use. Washington DC. National Academy Press, 1992.
36. Grimshaw JM, Russell IT. Effect of clinical guidelines on medical practice: a systemic review of rigorous evaluations. Lancet 1993;342(8883):1317-1322.
37. Abramson J. Overdo$ed America. Harper Perennial. New York 205, P127-128.
38. Pittet D, Hugonnet S, Harbarth S, Mourouga P, Sauvan V, Touveneau S, et al, and members of the Infection Control Programme. Effectiveness of a hospital-wide programme to improve compliance with handwashing. Lancet 2000;356(9238):1307-1312.

"Oh... look at this"

"Nursing would be a dream job if there were no doctors."
Gerhard Kocher

When I first started as an intensive care specialist, if a patient developed acute renal failure, an arterio-venous shunt would be inserted, a technician would wheel down a dialysis machine from the renal unit, the patient would be hooked-up to the machine and dialysed. The dialysis would continue for 3 to 6 hours every second or third day depending upon the degree of tissue breakdown in the critically ill patient. The technician would also regionally heparinise the patient (i.e. the blood would be anticoagulated when it entered the machine and reversed when it was reinfused back into the patient).

Continuous dialysis is now performed at the bedside by the intensive care nursing staff.

In America there are respiratory technicians who control the mechanical ventilator. They alter the inspired oxygen and all mechanical parameters that deliver gas into and out of the lungs (e.g. flow, volume and pressure of inspiratory and expiratory gases).

In Australasia the intensive care nurses perform these tasks.

In addition, ICU nurses monitor the arterial, venous, intracardiac and intracranial pressures, regularly perform respiratory suction, monitor arterial saturation, perform blood gas analysis, drain nasogastric and abdominal secretions, administer oral, intravenous and epidural medications, regularly change the patient's position in bed, perform mouth and eye toilet as well as write a report and talk to the relatives.

It is a busy and demanding day. Intensive care units would not exist without this specialised workforce. In the five units I have worked in, the majority of intensive care nurses were women, although an increasing number of men are now beginning to find fulfilment in this profession.

At the Flinders Medical Centre ICU during 2005 there were two morning ward rounds. The first began at 8:00 a.m. It was a 'handover' round where the night registrar presented the patients' active problems, their management during the night shift and their progress. This round often lasted 60 minutes but varied between 30 minutes and 2 hours. It would be interspersed with interruptions for new admissions and emergency procedures, where one or more specialists or trainees would leave to manage the acute problem. At the completion of this round the intensivists would often take a coffee break and retire to the anachronistically described 'tea-room'. We would always sit in our customary chairs and 'small talk' until the radiographic and biochemical tests were ready for the mid-morning 'image and biochem' round at 10:30 a.m.

On one occasion, the female senior nursing staff decided to inhabit our medical domain rather than theirs and have their social meeting 10 minutes before we arrived in 'our' tea-room for our morning coffee break.

The director of the ICU in sham rage blurted "what's this?"

"Nothing, Al – we just decided to use this room for our coffee break this morning," the nurse team leader replied.

"What?' said Al, still in character.

"We won't be long," was the nonchalant reply. The other nurses were starting to feel a little uncomfortable in continuing this provocative confrontation, whereas the other intensivists who were standing just inside the door watching this performance were all grinning.

"Well...." said Al, throwing his hands about and looking at us in mock exasperation. By this time the nursing team leader was the only one left sitting, and in Al's chair at that – the other nurses had left their seats and were gradually filing out the door. Finally the team leader got out of the chair muttering, "we had just finished anyway. You can have the room now!"

"Oh... look at this," said Al "we have Candida now all over the seats." He began to frantically brush the seat of his chair with his hand.

"Al, you can't say that!" I said, starting to chuckle. The rest of the medical staff were no help; they were all howling with laughter.

L. I. G. Worthley

The nursing team leader gently shook her head and left with a smile on her face.

Al continued to dust all the chairs until the nursing staff had left. He then began to smile.

The *esprit de corps* was strong between medical and nursing staff at the Flinders Medical Centre. If there was any genuine trouble between nursing and medical staff, it was always dealt with 'in house' and to everybody's satisfaction. If the issues remained unresolved there was always the ability for nurses or medical staff to report their problems to hospital administration, but I must say I cannot recall this ever happening.

Section 2. On death and dying

"... and needs to be admitted to the ICU"

"Medicine knows no limits, especially not its own."
Gerhard Kocher

A referral to an intensive care unit means a referral to an intensivist. A call by a junior doctor in a busy public hospital with a statement "Mrs. Jones is a day three post-op intestinal bypass patient who's had an excellent surgical result, but is now hypoxic and hypotensive and needs to be admitted to the ICU", does not fulfil the criteria for admission to the ICU – it is a request for an opinion. Intensive care units by themselves do not cure patients.

I trudged up the stairs to a surgical floor late one Friday evening after one such telephone request where a patient, who had been hypotensive and oligo-anuric for the previous 18 hours, had developed progressive hypoxia. She had been heparinised for a suspected pulmonary embolism (although the spiral CT earlier that day revealed only bilateral basal consolidation and effusions), given intravenous meropenem 500 mg 8-hourly for a suspected pneumonia and was currently being infused with the 8th litre of 0.9% saline.

She had type 2 diabetes with a past history of ischaemic heart disease. The operation three days ago was a small bowel bypass for intestinal obstruction caused by peritoneal dissemination of an ovarian carcinoma. Her liver function tests showed moderate elevation of the enzymes alanine aminotransferase, aspartate aminotransferase and alkaline phosphatase and her plasma creatinine was 0.28 mmol/L. The arterial blood gases revealed a PaO_2 of 55 mmHg, $PaCO_2$ 42 mmHg and pH 7.18 with an arterial lactate of 6.6 mmol/L. The chest X-ray confirmed the bilateral basal consolidation and effusions, and now revealed generalised pulmonary interstitial and alveolar infiltrates.

All of this I gleaned from the case notes, the attending nurse and the treatment sheet. The junior medical officer, with whom I had a cursory conversation some 10 minutes ago, had signed off on the week's work and was nowhere to be found.

The patient was in a side room surrounded by a bevy of concerned relatives. An oxygen mask sat awkwardly over her mouth and appeared to hinder rather than help her breathing. Her cheeks were sunken and her eyes were closed. All who surrounded her turned to me when I entered the room.

"G'day," I said, trying to sound 'homely' as I scanned the room. "I'm Doctor Worthley, an intensive care specialist. I've been asked to see Mrs. Jones."

I focused on the man who was at her side and said "You must be her . . . ?" waiting for him to fill in the gap, as I have been caught before by saying 'husband' when it was the son, friend, brother or, these days 'partner'.

"Husband" he said firmly.

"I wonder if you would excuse me then, while I look at your good wife." I said gesturing to the door. "I will see you in about 15 minutes or so in the relatives' room, which is at the end of the corridor."

One by one the family gradually left the room. I closed the door behind them so I could be left in peace with the patient. Mrs. Jones opened her eyes slowly at the commotion.

"You've probably had better days," I said, trying to put her at ease. She gave me half a smile and shrugged. With each breath her nostrils flared and a deep expiratory rattle could be heard. Her pupils were pinpoint. The morphine was having an effect.

"Have you any pain at the moment?" I enquired, beginning my formal assessment.

I continued with many other questions that required largely 'yes' or 'no' answers, as I knew she was finding it difficult to concentrate. I finished by saying that I would return after I had talked to her husband.

I wandered down the corridor knowing that her respiratory failure was caused by bilateral pulmonary consolidation, pleural effusions and pulmonary oedema, much of which had been caused by sputum retention, sepsis and excess 0.9% saline. Her hypotension was also due to sepsis, which was probably caused by an acute abdominal disorder (e.g. leaking anastomosis, ischaemic or infarcted bowel) as she had diffuse abdominal tenderness. However, despite the initial description by the referring doctor of a patient who had 'an excellent surgical result', I felt sure that the surgical team would not re-operate on my clinical interpretation.

"Ah, Mr. Jones" I said "I wonder if I could have a brief word with you," and ushered him away from the rest of his family to a small room close by.

"I have looked at your wife and reviewed her notes. Unfortunately, both her heart and lungs are failing following her operation, and I have been asked to review her concerning the possibility of managing her in intensive care on 'life support.'"

"You know she's got cancer, Doc," was his curt reply.

"Yes...." I said, measuring my response, as I wished him to continue.

"Before the operation she said that she was probably going to die. Now after the operation she is in continual pain," he said, burying his head in his hands. He then looked up and with a degree of frustration and anger said "She just wants to be left alone with her family, Doc."

I paused just long enough before I responded, to ensure he knew that what I said would not be just a cliché.

"I can understand that." I smiled and paused again. "In intensive care, we do have equipment that can keep patients alive while treatment such as surgery may be given time to be effective, yet we are not in the business of prolonging death if there is no hope." I waited for a response. He gazed at the wall and remained silent.

"Has she said what she would want to happen if she required 'life support' therapy?" I asked, attempting to open up the question of palliation.

"Oh, she has made it quite clear, Doc, she doesn't want to be kept alive if there's no hope. She only agreed to this operation when the doctors said that once they bypassed her cancer she could expect to live for up to a year or more in good health."

"A year or more?" I said not trying to sound surprised. I thought that the surgical team would perhaps say an optimistic 'three to six months' to the question of: 'How long do you think the patient would live if the surgery is successful?' I didn't think that they would suggest 'a year or more'. In my estimate, she would be lucky to survive more than a few weeks - less, if the diagnosis of an acute abdomen was right.

"A year or more," I repeated, still trying to hide my disbelief. "Well, at the moment, if nothing is done she will not survive the next 24 hours. Even if we admit her to intensive care and put her on 'life support', we may only just prolong her death."

Mr. Jones did not flinch. He had been direct with me, so I was direct with him.

"Doc, you have a talk to her. She does not want any useless meddling" he said, and stood as if to mark the end of our conversation.

I returned to Mrs. Jones and realised that after a few simple questions, intensive care and its technology was not what she wanted. She knew that she was dying, there was no bitterness towards the medical profession, she just wanted to be left in comfort, if not at home then at hospital, with her family, until she died.

I managed to contact the consultant who performed the intestinal bypass, and informed him that Mrs. Jones declined the help of intensive care and wished only to be kept comfortable. I had the impression that he was grateful that I had discussed the issues of dying with his patient, but probably would have preferred me to have admitted her to intensive care to manage her palliation.

As I returned to my office I wondered about the future for intensivists. Will we become responsible for all end-of-life decisions and management of patients who have not responded to medical or surgical treatment and who require palliative care?

I suddenly began thinking about my retirement.

"While we often manage dying patients, dying is not an indication for admission to an ICU"

"From inability to let well alone; from too much zeal for the new and contempt for what is old; from putting knowledge before wisdom, science before art, and cleverness before common sense; from treating patients as cases; and from making the cure of the disease more grievous than the endurance of the same, Good Lord deliver us."
Robert Hutchison

He was 87 years old with a past history of tuberculosis, bronchiectasis and severe ischaemic heart disease. His ischaemic heart disease had left him with a dilated cardiomyopathy which required hospitalisation on numerous occasions, particularly over the last six months, due to episodes of acute pulmonary oedema. This admission was no different. He normally had a chronic cough but it had become worse during the night, finally leaving him distraught and gasping for breath. He had previously declared that he did not want cardiopulmonary resuscitation (CPR) in the event of a cardiac arrest, so he was admitted to a general ward for comfort care. However, the 'not for CPR' message had not been relayed to the nursing staff so a cardiac arrest call was activated when he became unconscious and pulseless. Intubation, ventilation, 300mg of amiodarone intravenously, two shocks and he was back in sinus rhythm. The cardiac arrest team burst through the door of the intensive care unit, unannounced, and presented us with an obtunded and intubated patient. It was only when we read his notes that the background of this man's problems and his wishes emerged.

Thankfully, he was able to be extubated within the next few hours. We monitored him for a further 24 hours and discharged him to the 'home' team for further management. During the next few days he remained oxygen dependent with resistant pulmonary oedema and worsening renal failure, and was admitted to the coronary care unit for further management.

During the period in coronary care, the idea that an aspiration pneumonia was the predominant problem gained momentum.

"If it's just a pneumonia, we could anaesthetise him and put him on a breathing machine to enable us to remove the sputum which will then allow him to get better," the junior cardiology registrar eagerly informed the family. "So we will ask the ICU team to admit him. They could also dialyse him."

As the intensive care registrar was a little unsure of my view on this new turn in events, he asked me my opinion before admitting the patient to the intensive care unit.

"Do you remember Mr. Smith, the man with a dilated cardiomyopathy who was 'not for CPR' but was resuscitated and admitted to ICU for 24 hours after he had a cardiac arrest?" the ICU registrar began.

"Yes" I said.

"Well the cardiac registrar said that he needs to come to intensive care for a short period of mechanical ventilation and dialysis to tide him over his aspiration pneumonia and renal failure."

"Really!" I replied. I imagine I probably had a wry smile on my face. "I better have a look at him then."

I first reviewed Mr. Smith's case notes to see what had occurred over the last few days and if he had rescinded his decision to not undergo CPR or 'life support therapy' in the event of a cardiac or respiratory arrest. His recent investigations revealed that there had been no change in his temperature, pulse, chest X-ray or white cell count, and a repeated echocardiogram still demonstrated an ejection fraction of 15% with biventricular dilation and left ventricular global hypokinesis.

I went to his bedside and reintroduced myself. "Good morning Mr. Smith, I am Dr. Worthley, you may remember me. I was the ICU specialist who managed you a few days ago."

He was drowsy and breathless but nodded in acknowledgement. I added "I'm sorry to see that you still have trouble with your breathing. Do you mind if I have a look at you?"

He nodded his head slightly and closed his eyes, so I began. I looked at his breathing pattern, asked him to take a deep breath, hold it and then cough, and then listened to his chest. He had coarse crepitations throughout both lung fields and gross peripheral oedema. The pulse oximeter revealed a saturation varying between 86% and 88% whilst breathing oxygen through a facemask.

After asking the registrar to hold my stethoscope, I held the patient's hand and said slowly, "Mr. Smith, we have been asked to look at the possibility of giving you life support therapy." I stopped for a moment to allow him to concentrate on what I was saying. "However, I remember that you did not want this the last time we met. Have you changed your mind?"

He opened his eyes a little, looked at me and shook his head. I looked at the ICU registrar and said, "I think I should talk to the relatives."

During a discussion with the patient's son and two daughters, I stated that their father's predominant problem remained his severe cardiac failure and that aspiration pneumonia was not an important component of his illness. Furthermore, as he confirmed that he did not want life support therapy, his treatment should be concerned with ensuring that he remained comfortable.

I documented this in the patient's notes, phoned the cardiac team to state that this man did not have an aspiration pneumonia, did not want ICU life support, required an improvement in his current conservative treatment, and that perhaps morphine may be useful. I then turned to the intensive care trainee and said that any request that includes the statement 'the patient needs to come to intensive care' is really an intensive care consult. I added, "it's pretty simple: intensivists are responsible for the admission and discharge policies for the ICU. If we believe that the ICU and its staff have the facilities and expertise that will benefit the patient, the patient should be admitted, otherwise admission is not required. While we often manage dying patients, dying is not an indication for admission to an ICU."

L. I. G. Worthley

The patient died three days later.

The dying patient

Because I could not stop for death –
He kindly stopped for me –
The carriage held but just ourselves –
And immortality.
   Emily Dickinson

   No disease is fatal until the patient dies, so one can only diagnose a disease as fatal in retrospect. Nevertheless, there are some diseases where survival is not only unexpected but also unprecedented.
   The late Elisabeth Kübler-Ross, in her book, 'On Death and Dying' described five stages of grieving experienced by the dying patient (i.e. denial, anger, bargaining, depression and acceptance). These stages may also be detected in the relatives of a critically ill patient. However, the stages of denial and anger are the most common and most challenging for the intensivist to manage. Ms Kübler-Ross stated "the more we are making advancements in science, the more we seem to fear and deny the reality of death"; yet it is as natural to be born as it is to die.
   With current technology, death in the intensive care unit is often perceived to be an extraordinary event, as if respiratory or cardiopulmonary arrests are predictable and reversible. While it is acknowledged that an eternal mortal life is impossible, a grieving relative tends to be oblivious to this fact, denying the reality that death of their loved one may be imminent and that the intensive care unit may simply be prolonging this process.
   One such patient was admitted to the intensive care unit with a history of sudden respiratory failure following a mild upper respiratory tract infection. The husband assiduously followed his wife, who had been intubated in the emergency room, up to the ICU floor and watched as the nursing staff established her on the mechanical ventilator, placed the cardiac monitoring leads on her chest, connected the intravascular lines and began the standard medical observations.

"How long has she been unwell?" I asked her nervous husband.

"Only about 3 to 4 days" he said, "Is she going to be all right?"

"She's in the best place possible and we will give her every opportunity to get better," I replied. I asked him about her previous medical condition, as we had no prior medical record of her being admitted to our hospital.

"She's been reasonably well and had no previous medical problems to talk about. And apart from the birth of our children, this is her first admission to hospital," was his reply, which seemed unusual as the patient's inspiratory pressure, with normal ventilatory settings, seemed to be abnormally high. Also, the sputum was thin and white and the chest X-ray revealed a generalized granular pattern, all of which seemed to indicate an underlying chronic respiratory problem.

We continued her management over the ensuing days with no typical or atypical respiratory infective agent being detected and little change in her respiratory status. On the eighth day it was decided that we would need to do a tracheostomy to facilitate further management.

At this stage we had only seen her husband. There were two children, a daughter who was a single mother, who lived in the country and was unable to see her mother due to the needs of her young family, and a son who was on business in some remote part of China.

Finally, on the weekend before we were about to perform the tracheostomy, the daughter arrived. We quickly ushered her into the room to see her mother.

"She looks at peace, doctor. But why is she on the breathing machine?" The patient's husband began to fidget.

I explained that as she had been previously fit and well we had to do everything possible to return her to good health.

"But she has been a respiratory cripple for the last five years. She normally sees Dr. Hall at the Queen Elizabeth Hospital for chronic fibrotic lung disease. She has had numerous hospital admissions and been admitted twice to intensive care. Dad now manages her at home in bed with a constant oxygen supply. She expressly wished not to be resuscitated if she stops breathing."

I was shocked, I turned to the husband and said "But . . . ." He suddenly held his head in his hands and began to weep.

Inside God's Shed

"I knew that if I told you that, you would not have treated her and she would have died," he sobbed. Over the next few days and with the help of the daughter and the local priest, the patient was allowed to die in peace with the husband at her side and constantly informed about the process.

Once, medical paternalism may have been an important part in the management of termination of life; now, however it is unacceptable. Moreover, to say that what we are doing is 'not in the patient's best interest' can often confuse family members as it would seem to them a fatuous comment, one without meaning, as the patient and family has no 'interest' in death. Even in the presence of a living will, while in theory the relatives' wishes do not have the power to dictate treatment, clinicians commonly look to the family for guidance, as common experience (and legal resolutions) indicate that it is unwise to ignore the family's views. Finally, there is no judgment more dangerous than that someone else's life (given the age, illness and underlying past history of the patient) is not worth living. It is an unacceptable concept to both a loving family and a caring physician.

Some ethicists have argued that the question of withholding or removal of life support should be decided on the basis of what the person would have wanted for him or her self, before the condition declared itself. However, it is often unknown for certain what a person would have wanted before the condition declared itself. Also, what a person wants can change as his or her circumstances change. Quadriplegics who unexpectedly wish to continue to live illustrate one of the dangers of making a living will. Yet there will be a state in which the continuation of life is a torment rather than a blessing, and skilled medical staff can usually recognise the inevitability of death in these terminally ill patients.

For the clinician treating the dying patient and their relatives, methods to steer a calm and reasoned course through the 'end of life' stages are not simple.

Right to die, withdrawal of therapy and the ICU as a medical purgatory

"I am ready to meet my maker. Whether my maker is prepared for the ordeal of meeting me is another matter."
    Winston Churchill

I knew that it was going to be a long day. It was the Monday morning round. The intensive care unit was full, nursing staff were racing around shouting orders at each other, telling me to cancel the cardiothoracic list 'because we had no beds'. The night resident began the hand over by stating that the first patient who had just been admitted, intubated, ventilated and paralysed, was an 81 year old man who had 'terminal' emphysema. He had had numerous hospital admissions for acute-on-chronic respiratory failure and had been oxygen dependent for the last 12 months. His most recent hospital admission was two and a half months ago, requiring a three-week period of mechanical ventilation and a prolonged convalescence in hospital. When he was finally discharged home he remained breathless and bed-bound. He had given strict instructions to his only daughter, with whom he lived, to ensure that the next time he was admitted he was not to be put on 'life support' again. What happened?

It seemed that the daughter found her father unconscious after returning home from a brief shopping trip. She called an ambulance and arrived with him at hospital to be asked by an accident and emergency resident "do you want your father to be treated actively?" She was unmarried and had been his carer for the past 5 years, her life revolved around him. He wasn't a burden to her; indeed she had enjoyed 'mothering' him. To the question 'do you want your father to be treated actively?' her response could only be "of course I do. I want you to do everything possible." The ICU registrar was contacted and informed, "Remember Mr. X? Well, he's back again and his relatives want every thing to be done." The die was cast - thiopentone, suxamethonium, intubation, all in A&E, and pancuronium 12 mg i.v. 'to stabilise him for the trip to ICU'.

The rest of the ICU ward round was somewhat simpler. The remaining four patients who had been admitted overnight had problems that resolved rapidly, and could be discharged to the care of their home team. The 'cardiacs' could now be accommodated, and there was less shouting by the ICU nursing staff. I asked the ICU registrar if she could organise the discharge of patients who were admitted overnight so that I could sit and have a chat with Mr X's daughter.

The daughter was rational and reasoned. She understood that her father's wishes had been contravened; yet when asked 'do you want your father to be treated actively?' she stated that she could not bring herself to make the decision to stop treatment.

I began by saying that her father was sedated and comfortable at the moment and we were continuing to ensure that he remained so. However, there was no treatment available that would return him back to health. Her father knew this, and as his life was coming to a close it appeared that it was also becoming unbearable. If he required resuscitation, he had expressed a wish not be put on 'life support'. We did not have to make a decision; the decision had already been made by him. By withholding or withdrawing 'life support' we would simply be carrying out this wish. I stated it was unfortunate that she had been confronted by a clumsy question of 'do you want your father to be treated actively?' because we treated everybody actively. We would provide all that was necessary to allow him a comfortable death. Currently, what we were doing was simply prolonging his death.

The daughter felt comfortable with the fact that her father would be taken from the respirator and provided with a peaceful end. She understood that we were adhering to his wishes and was relieved to find she was not required to personally authorise his demise.

Nobody seems to die any more; they have cardiac or respiratory arrests, and arrive in the ICU for further management. Perhaps it is because intensive care medicine has promoted itself as a discipline that can reverse any illness? Perhaps futility can now only be defined by the intensivist? While the right to refuse treatment remains the patient's prerogative, who is going to be sued if the patient is brought into hospital, unconscious and against their wishes by their family?

Withdrawal or withholding treatment is an important part of the intensivist's practice and in some ICU's accounts for up to 90% of all deaths.[1] It is performed if the patient is brain dead, if the patient (or surrogate) refuses or withdraws consent for life support therapy, or medical treatment is deemed futile and simply prolongs suffering and an inevitable end.[2,3,4,5,6,7,8]

Brain death can be established relatively easily when standard criteria are met.[9] The relatives can be informed with absolute certainty that consciousness is lost forever.[10] However, the commonest reason for withdrawal or withholding therapy in the ICU is futility of treatment in the terminally ill patient,[11] although the reasons of futility and the patient's right to refuse treatment are often interwoven.

Concerning the right to refuse life support therapy; by the time the patient requires intensive care, unless a previous declaration has been made, they are usually incapable of making medical decisions. The family is often asked to articulate the patient's wishes, concerning the continuation of treatment.[12] In this regard, the relatives should not be asked whether they would want treatment continued or withheld, but in the knowledge of what is wrong, what the therapeutic options are and what the prognosis is, whether they believe that the patient would want 'life support' to be continued or withheld.[12]

Concerning futility, despite the numerous multivariable intensive care scoring systems that have been proposed in an attempt to accurately determine the outcome of a critically ill patient, the predictive abilities of the currently used scoring systems are not accurate enough to make them prognostically useful. All continue to show a failure rate of 15 - 20% in predicting the outcome in individual patients.[13] For the moment, good clinical judgement guided by experience appears to be just as accurate.

Futility has both quantitative (i.e. likelihood of achieving a final outcome) and qualitative (i.e. likelihood that final outcome will be acceptable to the patient) aspects.[14] One has to gauge the likelihood of survival as well as quality of survival when talking to the family. Yet, while futility should only be judged on likelihood of achieving a desired outcome, in practice other factors often influence the decision to withdraw therapy. For example clinicians tend to withdraw therapy if the organ failure has developed naturally rather than iatrogenically, or withdrawal results in an immediate death or in a delayed death if the diagnosis is uncertain.[15]

Although it is inappropriate to offer futile treatment to the patient,[16] the process of withdrawal of therapy is a sensitive issue and usually only occurs when the family has come to terms with the prognosis. One response to dealing with a request for futile treatment (e.g. cardiopulmonary resuscitation) is to practice a 'slow code' (e.g. to go through the motions of performing cardiopulmonary resuscitation with the aim and hope that the patient will not survive). However this 'sham' simply provides a prolonged and painful death in an attempt to satisfy distressed patients or relatives. It has no justification.[17] With honesty, goodwill and close communication with all concerned, the decision to withdraw therapy will generally be reached with time.[16]

Once the decision has been reached, the relatives often ask 'how long will it take?', 'can I be with him/her when he/she dies?' and 'will there be any pain or distress?'

To determine 'how long will it take' requires experience, and it is best to give a tolerably wide range, without losing the confidence of the family. If the patient is mechanically ventilated with a high inspired oxygen and high catecholamine requirement, one may reasonably state that it should not take long (and when pressed perhaps 10 to 20 minutes). I often state that the patient may die immediately or linger for hours, as we ensure that they are comfortable without actively hastening death. Similarly, withdrawal of ventilation from a post cardiac arrest patient who after three days is still deeply unconscious may result in a patient who is able to breathe quietly and comfortably for days before finally succumbing to hypoxia from sputum retention and bronchopneumonia.

'Can I be with him/her when he/she dies?' I find can only be answered with a 'sure', as any other response tends to be regarded suspiciously. I tend to follow it up with 'but you must realise that a dying patient can be a grim if not hideous sight.' I then outline some reflex changes that they may observe, so that they are fully aware of what to expect if these changes do occur (e.g. blue grey appearance, 'gurgling' breath sounds, eye opening and looking upwards, spinal reflexes of arm or leg movements, even opisthotonos i.e. severe arching of the back).

Finally, withdrawal of life support is not an abandonment of the patient, and to the question 'will there be any pain or distress?', the answer must be that we will do all we can to relieve any suffering.[18]

Withdrawal of therapy is an important part of the intensivist's activity yet it is rarely taught, often performed awkwardly or ignored with the ICU becoming a medical purgatory filled with patients who are 'treated to death'. Like all aspects of medical therapy, its management requires honesty, frankness, trust and a genuine concern for all who are involved. If it is regarded as a chore to simply 'tidy up' the ICU, lawyers will be called in.

REFERENCES
1. Karlawish JHT, Hall JB. Managing death and dying in the intensive care unit. Am J Resp Crit Care Med 1997;155:1-2.
2. Task Force on Ethics of the Society of Critical Care Medicine. Consensus report on the ethics of foregoing life-sustaining treatments in the critically ill. Crit Care Med 1990;18:1435-1439.
3. Tomlinson T, Brody H. Ethics and communication in do-not-resuscitate orders. N Engl J Med 1988;318:43-46.
4. Ruark JE, Raffin TA, and the Stanford University Medical Center Committee on Ethics. Initiating and withdrawing life support. Principles and practice in adult medicine. N Engl J Med 1988;318:25-30.
5. Smedira NG, Evans BH, Grais LS, Cohen NH, Lo B, Cooke M, et al. Withholding and withdrawal of life support from the critically ill. N Engl J Med 1990;32:309-315.
6. Blackhall LJ. Must we always use CPR? N Engl J Med 1987;317:1281-1285.
7. Jennett B. Decisions to limit treatment. Lancet 1987;2(8562):787-788.
8. Luce JM. Conflicts over ethical principles in the intensive care unit. Crit Care Med 1992;20:313-315.

9. Conference of Medical Royal Colleges and their Faculties (UK). Diagnosis of brain death. Br Med J 1976;ii:1187-1188.
10. Pallis C. Reappraising death. Br Med J 1982;285:1409-1412.
11. Prendergast TJ, Luce JM. Increased incidence of withholding and withdrawal of life support from the critically ill. Am J Resp Crit Care Med 1997;155:15-20.
12. Luce JM, Fink C. Communicating with families about withholding and withdrawal of life support. Chest 1992;101:1185-1186.
13. Kirby RR, Civetta JM. Critical care. In: Brown DL, ed. Outcome in anesthesia. Philadelphia: JP Lippincott, 1988:184.
14. Jecker NS, Pearlman RA. Medical futility. Who decides? Arch Intern Med 1992;152:1140-1144.
15. Christakis NA, Asch DA. Biases in how physicians choose to withdraw life support. Lancet 1993;342(8872):642-646.
16. Snider GL. Withholding and withdrawing life-sustaining therapy. All systems are not yet "go". Am J Resp Crit Care Med 1995;151:279-281.
17. Gazelle G. The slow code - should anyone rush to its defense? N Engl J Med 1998;338:467-469.
18. Brody H, Campbell ML, Faber-Langendoen K, Ogle KS. Withdrawing intensive life-sustaining treatment - recommendations for compassionate clinical management. N Engl J Med 1997;336:652-657.

Critical care medicine and its cost

"Care is never futile, but medical interventions sometimes are."
Leah Curtin[1]

The ICU patient demographic is changing with the increase in age being the most obvious shift. The proportion of intensive care unit hours dedicated to patients aged over 80 is increasing by 15% per annum. Patients are now sicker and their expectations are greater; in some cases unrealistically so. When dealing with a critically ill patient the clinician does not focus on cost of treatment *per se* but on making the patient better, even though the common wisdom suggests that any treatment that is 'second rate' is also economically wasteful.

There will always be ways that one can improve the patient's care by spending more money; however hospital administrators do not have an unrestricted budget and health funding is not limitless despite the professed aim of the World Health Organisation of 'health for all by the year 2000'.

While, in theory, clinicians should administer the highest quality of care at the cheapest price, defining what is the highest quality of care attainable at the cheapest price will always be difficult. What often begins as the best medicine at the lowest price sooner or later becomes an obsession with cost, as cost can be easily measured whereas 'best medicine' cannot. So it becomes medical care that is 'in accordance with good clinical practice' provided at the lowest cost (i.e. what is politically tolerable).

The facts concerning the cost of acute medical care include: 1) medical costs are rising faster than the cost of living, 2) 50% of a hospital budget is spent on the last 6 weeks of life, and 3) more than 70% - 80% of the hospital budget is used for wages. Therefore, to reduce hospital costs, doctors and nurses need to be fired.

The sick patient is not an economic person. He or she is ignorant, fearful, helpless, miserable, and wanting health at almost any price. They want the doctor to consider their problems with no other thought other than how to best restore his or her health. They want no second best and certainly do not want his or her needs weighed against the claims of other patients. The patient, in brief, is looking for a 'trustee' not a 'provider' and as such wants to be considered as a beneficiary not a consumer. The clinician also wants to be able to discharge this trust as effectively as possible without being influenced by matters of over servicing.

However, public expectations of the hospital system continually change. In the 1960's to receive long-term mechanical ventilation (i.e. 'life support') a patient had to have had a knighthood, a career, a loving family and a friend on the hospital board. Today a heartbeat is sufficient. Interestingly, people who pay nothing towards the cost of their care make substantially heavier demands on health services than those who do. Total expenditure rises steadily as payment by the user falls.[2] Concerning these expectations and use of the intensive care unit, 'not for cardiopulmonary resuscitation', 'not for invasive ventilation' and withdrawal of therapy are now becoming harder and harder to direct. Despite careful and considered discussion, some remain suspicious and believe that financial triage and not futility determine the use of CPR or 'life support'.

The patient's relatives often expect unrestricted access to health services and believe that it is 'their right' to have this service, demanding the use of 'futile' support and unattainable results. If these expectations are unfulfilled they are now likely to consult their lawyers, and do so even though there is evidence to show that clinicians are becoming better qualified, better trained and more conscious of malpractice. Intensive care is a growth industry.

One of the freedoms of our society is that we are allowed to make our own judgement in what we wish to be foolish about when it comes to spending our own money. However, when health issues are at stake, it seems that we are able to be foolish about spending other people's money as well. Hospitals provide care for millions of people who cannot pay. The poor may be denied social service of shelter and food yet they are not denied an operation and intensive care services that can cost thousands of dollars.

All this indicates that the intensive care community (i.e. physicians and nurses) must communicate and inform the public of the realities of life-threatening diseases, the influence of co-morbidities and the benefit, or otherwise, of prolonged life support. We offer treatment that can cure but in the event of unremitting disease we can not offer miracles.

REFERENCES
1. Curtin L. Patient wishes and futile interventions. Healthcare Traveler April 1, 2005. (http://healthcaretraveler.modernmedicine .com)
2. Editorial. The Rand Health Insurance Study: a spanner in the works? Lancet 1986;1(8488):1012-1013.

Section 3. Teaching and research

"I touch the future. I teach"[1]

"Those of us who have the duty of training the rising generation of doctors . . . must not inseminate the virgin minds of the young with the tares of our own fads . . . . It is always well, before handing the cup of knowledge to the young, to wait until the froth has settled."
Robert Hutchison

Medicine has a long and distinguished history of teachers. The word *'doctor'* has been derived from the Latin word *'doctoris'* meaning teacher. Three hundred years BC the Greek physician Hippocrates declared "I will impart this Art by precept, by lecture and by every mode of teaching, not only to my own sons but to the sons of those who taught me and to disciples bound by the covenant and oath, according to the Law of Medicine." William Osler said "I desire no other epitaph . . . than the statement that I taught medical students in the wards, as I regard this as by far the most useful and important work I have been called upon to do."

Nevertheless, I really didn't like undergraduate teaching. The students were young and sweaty and more interested in the weekend social events than my lectures. It wasn't so much their large rings through the lobes of both ears or neck tattoos that worried me particularly (although if they graduated I wondered how their patients would react to them), it was the disinterested shrug of their shoulders when I asked questions that bothered me. They gave me the distinct impression that they wanted to be spoon fed with all the answers; no thinking, no effort, no thanks.

I started to feel sorry for the teachers of my own undergraduate years. Surely I wasn't that bad. Perhaps I was. I remember thinking more about one of the George Harrison riffs in 'Drive my car' during a combined 4th year and 6th year student lecture on renal failure when I was suddenly asked by the lecturer "What is the most important clinical investigation in renal disease?" I was abruptly returned to reality.

"Ah . . . " I said, and before I could collect myself he added,

"Oh, you're a 4th year medical student then, sorry." He was about to turn to another student when I replied – and with regret,

"Err . . . No. I'm a 6th year medical student."

Without hesitating and without a smile he stage whispered,

"First time then?" the class burst out laughing.

He wanted me to say "urinalysis." A 4th year medical student next to me offered the correct answer as soon as the class settled.

Postgraduate teaching was another matter. I loved it. You 'touch the future'.[1] The students were a mature age group who had mortgages and children. They were incredibly motivated to learn as much as they could about the specialty of intensive care medicine; to graduate, become a specialist – and pay off the mortgage. Whether at the bedside or in the classroom, the postgraduate trainee would appreciate both teaching forums. At the bedside they would keenly watch as I examined a patient. What could be demonstrated? Why was it important? Were the signs useful? Were the signs evidence-based? We would discuss all things long and hard. I hoped to provide a method from the history and physical examination that would work for the critically ill patient and allow the trainee to diagnose the most likely disorder, before embarking on the confirmatory tests. The students came prepared, so the session taught them how to problem solve and how to diagnose and manage the patient. The students would already have a broad knowledge of medicine. I was simply there to help them how to think, not what to think. I provided many handouts, which were finally published in three monographs.[2,3,4]

During my 40-year professional life my research was predominantly in small clinical trials of minor importance. It was in my teaching that I derived my most satisfying experiences.

REFERENCES
1. Hohler, Robert T. I Touch the Future: The Story of Christa McAuliffe. New York, NY: Random House, 1986
2. Worthley LIG. Clinical examination of the critically ill patient, 3rd Ed. Melbourne: The Australasian Academy of Critical Care Medicine, 2006.
3. Worthley LIG. Synopsis of Intensive Care Medicine. London: Churchill Livingstone, 1994.
4. Worthley LIG. Handbook of Emergency Laboratory Tests. New York: Churchill Livingstone 1996.

Cognitive development of the intensivist

"A good question is never answered. It is not a bolt to be tightened into place but a seed to be planted and to bear more seed toward the hope of greening the landscape of the idea."
   John Ciardi

   "Well how come everybody else does one thing and you do another?" one smart-alec trainee at the back of the room retorted, bringing a chuckle from the class.
   "Well, I have not found that," I responded. "All my informed colleagues seem to do what I do. You see if a thousand people decide to do a dumb thing it doesn't alter the fact that the decision is still a dumb one."
   It had been a long day; I was tired and was trying to get the class to review their practice on the use of inotropic agents (e.g. adrenaline, noradrenaline, dopamine) - what was the evidence? Do they reduce mortality? Unfortunately, I had now surrendered to the primitive instinct of repartee.
   I gathered my thoughts. "What I am trying to do is to teach you to think. That means: not doing what I do, not doing what other people do, but doing what you should do after careful consideration of all data. Always question dogma!" The class looked disinterested, they wanted commandments, and thinking appeared to be just too hard.

   The session finally came to a close. After more than 30 years teaching intensive care trainees, this was my last tutorial. To some extent I was relieved, although I was still left wondering about the cognitive development of the intensivist. How should one teach intensive care trainees? What is the difference between brain-washing and reasoning?
   While critically ill patients may present with a simple system failure, they often have complex clinical problems. The disease may appear to be straight-forward (e.g. acute respiratory distress syndrome,

acute renal failure), yet the underlying cause may be one of many (e.g. aspiration, pancreatitis, gut perforation, etc) and the patient may have many co-morbidities (e.g. diabetes, chronic renal failure, cirrhosis, chronic obstructive pulmonary disease, disseminated adenocarcinoma, etc). It seems to me that there is a compelling need to have the management of these patients carefully considered.

The novice intensive care trainee is often prone to protocolise patient management. Uncertainty, particularly early in their career, is not tolerated, and there are guidelines for shock, acute respiratory failure, oliguria and the like. To them there are either right (good) or wrong (bad) decisions.[1] Treatment is easy. Just follow the arrows, or using today's vernacular, 'connect the dots'.

However, inevitably they find that decisions often need to be made in the face of uncertainty and patients do not always respond as they should to the various algorithms.[1,2] Ultimately, the early dualistic (right/wrong) approach, gives way to the realisation that there may be more than one way to successfully manage a critically ill patient. Moreover, trainees soon discover that their mentors and 'landmark' articles are not infallible. Facts change. Eternal truths appear to be elusive.

Despite using the same body of evidence in databases (e.g. MEDLINE and the Cochrane Library), recommendations on the same disease often differ as the data can be interpreted in many different ways.[3,4] Often the differences in opinion of those writing guidelines from the 'evidence' relates to the extent to which the evidence obtained from selected populations of patients can be extrapolated to the general population. There may also be hidden biases (even from specialists in evidence-based medicine) that only emerge with provocation.[5]

Medicine is a probabilistic science that sometimes exhibits elements of chaos with the behaviour of disease and its response to therapy unable to be predicted exactly.[3,6,7] Chaos describes a non-linear dynamic system with no absolute predictability, and has little utility for the practitioner, who needs some degree of predictability to manage patients. However, the non-predictability of chaos appears to be only important the longer one observes the system. While the effect of a butterfly wing in Rio may lead to a storm in New York, using this argument it seems that a similar occurrence in Rio may also alter the orbit of Pluto - but both must be over different periods of time. Over short periods one may predict events with reasonable certainty, using pragmatic rules and formulae. For example, when we resuscitate a patient we know that one litre of blood infused over 30 minutes will elevate the blood pressure in a hypovolaemic patient. However, we do not know what the effect will be after a fortnight, but does it matter? We frequently monitor and intervene to alter this system and avert disaster if, after time (in the above case), it looks as though the patient is becoming hypovolaemic again or, on the other hand, developing pulmonary oedema.

While the intensivist's cognitive, affective and psychomotor domains all need to be developed, the trainee has to be able to tolerate ambiguity, with an ability to explore more than one interpretation of the findings.

The teacher should also teach the trainee how to think and not what to think.

REFERENCES
1. Benbassat J, Cohen R. Clinical instruction and cognitive development of medical students. Lancet 1982;1(8263):95-97.
2. Garfield FB, Garfield JM. Clinical judgment and clinical practice guidelines. Int J Technol Assess Health Care 2000;16:1050-1060.
3. Burgers JS, van Everdingen JJE. Beyond the evidence in clinical guidelines. Lancet 2004;364(9432):392-393.
4. Raine R, Sanderson C, Hutchings A, Carter S, Larkin K, Black N. An experimental study of determinants of group judgments in clinical guideline development. Lancet 2004;364(9432):429-437.
5. Chalmers I. Human albumin administration in critically ill patients. I would not want an albumin transfusion. BMJ 1998;317:885.
6. Lake FR. Teaching on the run tips: doctors as teachers. MJA 2004;180:415-416.
7. Prideaux D, Alexander H, Bower A, Dacre J, Haist S, Jolly B, et al. Clinical teaching: maintaining an educational role for doctors in the new health environment. Med Educ 2000;34:820-826.

Are intensive care units self-sustaining?

"If you have an important point to make, don't try to be subtle or clever. Use a pile driver. Hit the point once. Then come back and hit it again. Then hit it a third time – a tremendous whack."
Winston Churchill

Finally, we had reached the last patient of our morning ward round – a round that had been interrupted by trying to accommodate a request for three beds for patients from cardiothoracic theatre, an accident and emergency department trauma call and a cardiac arrest. The night registrar looked somewhat relieved, as he knew that his shift was about to end. He quickly ushered us to the foot of the bed and began by telling us that the patient had been admitted for postoperative management following a defunctioning colostomy for a bowel obstruction caused by a rectal carcinoma. It was an elective admission, as the patient had been admitted previously to the intensive care unit about 2 weeks ago with shock and acute respiratory failure caused by an E. coli septicaemia.

I recalled the patient's former admission and remember thinking at the time that much of his respiratory failure had probably been caused by our junior medical trainee. He had prescribed a generous infusion of colloid and crystalloid solutions in an attempt to generate a mean arterial pressure of 85 mmHg; a pressure he deemed necessary to 'guarantee adequate perfusion and reduce the risk of acute renal failure'. I also recalled that after ceasing the morphine and midazolam infusion, reducing the mean arterial pressure lower limit to 65 mmHg and attaining a large negative fluid balance, the patient was able to be extubated successfully without developing acute renal failure, although 4 days had elapsed before this was achieved.

The rectal carcinoma associated with his E. coli septicaemia was diagnosed during his ICU stay. As the tumour was not obstructing the bowel lumen a course of radiotherapy, following his discharge from the ICU was planned to reduce the tumour mass before definitive surgery. However, during a 10-day delay in arranging radiotherapy, the lesion suddenly became an obstructive one so a defunctioning colostomy was performed and he was electively readmitted to the ICU postoperatively for further management.

The patient remained intubated throughout the night with an infusion of morphine and midazolam (50 mg of each in a 50 mL syringe) to settle him. The infusion initially ran at 4 mL/hr which was rapidly increased up to 10 mL/hr. A mean arterial blood pressure lower limit of 85 mmHg was again prescribed and 3.0 litres of 0.9% saline, 1.5 litres of 4% albumin in 0.9% saline, 1 litre of Gelofusine®, two units of blood, 850 mL of fresh frozen plasma and finally a noradrenaline infusion (increasing up to 25 µg/min) had been administered throughout the night. At the morning ward round the patient was on 100% oxygen and 15 cm H_2O of positive end expiratory pressure with a PaO_2 of 82 mmHg.

"A 'Swan' (Swan Ganz catheter) has not been inserted?" I inquired.

The night registrar looked around for some support from his colleagues. "Well… as there have been no controlled trials showing any benefit with right heart catheterisation, and some even indicating an increase in morbidity with its use, I guess I felt that it would be better to manage him without one," he responded.

"So you used blood pressure only to assess the adequacy, or otherwise, of the circulation?" I asked.

"Yes - along with urine output and other signs" he nodded.

"Such as?" I inquired.

"Capillary return, triple rhythm, pulmonary crepitations," he replied, nodding again.

It was the at end of a long ward round and I didn't wish to denigrate the importance of physical signs, particularly when they seemed to be so enthusiastically promoted by a junior registrar (especially as some of our medical trainees seem to manage patients from a biochemical result book and a radiological screen rather than from the bedside). Nevertheless, I felt compelled to travel a little further with the conversation.

"Has the stethoscope undergone a prospective, randomised and controlled trial?" I asked.

The registrar began to shuffle.

"What about the percussion hammer, tuning fork, ophthalmoscope or even the palpating hand?" I was on a roll, "and why a mean arterial pressure of 85 mmHg? Why not 105 mmHg?"

The registrar looked a little confused as he probably wondered why I was challenging the subject of physical signs, particularly as I often strongly endorsed the use of the clinical examination and tried in vain to reintroduce its benefits to the consciousness of trainees. Moreover, wasn't the maintenance of blood pressure important?

"Gentleman…and Madam," I uttered, as there was also a young female trainee in our midst who was desperately trying not to catch my eye.

"I am not anti-clinical examination, I am just anti-'knee-jerk' medicine, anti-thoughtless medicine, call it what you like. The circulation is not just about arterial pressure, it is about preload and flow. The 'Swan' is *our* instrument. We should be experts in its use and abuse. This patient has a bad case of iatrogenic pulmonary oedema and has had the misfortune of having it twice in 2 weeks!" I said in exasperation.

There was no reply. Indeed the only sound that could be heard was the gentle hiss of the ventilator.

I turned to the 'day' registrar and said "insert a 'Swan' and let me know the results" and left.

A right heart catheter (i.e. the 'Swan') was inserted revealing a wedge pressure of 28 mmHg, a cardiac output of 12.5 L/min and mixed venous oxygen saturation of 82%. The patient underwent another trial of re-emergence; ceasing the morphine and midazolam, reducing the mean arterial pressure lower limit to 65 mmHg and, with the help of frusemide, inducing a large negative fluid balance. The patient was subsequently extubated, although this time it required only 2 days.

As I related the story to my colleagues I remember lamenting the fact that it wasn't the Swan Ganz catheter that was at fault, it was unidimensional thinking and protocolised or 'knee jerk' medicine that were the new weapons of mass destruction. That evening my wife was more understanding saying that young trainees were there to be taught and they will make mistakes. As I looked at the bottom of my glass containing the last few drops of a Shiraz, I became somewhat pragmatic "Why should I complain?" I thought, "my job is assured."

"If you knew 20 years ago what ICU medicine would be like today, do you think that you would still choose to be an intensivist?"

"In the sufferer let me see only the human being."
Maimonides

It was a balmy evening with not a breath of wind. The setting was made even more celestial by the last rays of the setting sun filtering through the vine on my back fence and flickering a kaleidoscope of red, yellow and gold on the rendered wall behind us. John and I were resting after a long day of teaching at a short course on intensive care medicine and were attempting to unwind while sipping a light ale. We had been talking about the various trainees - their weaknesses - their strengths when suddenly he said,

"Tub, why did your lads do cardiology?"

"I guess because they liked it" I replied.

"Yeah . . . but why did they *not* do intensive care medicine. I mean, did you actively discourage them?"

As both John and I have had difficulties with public hospital administrators, I began by saying,

"I don't think that I actively discouraged or encouraged them - although I probably was happier that they chose a discipline that would not lock them into requiring a public hospital appointment to practice their specialty."

He drank his last mouthful of ale and leaned back. His eyes glazed a little as he looked at his empty bottle and then dismissed my remarks with,

"Yeah, but all specialists usually try to get a public hospital appointment and probably have as much trouble as we do with administration."

He sucked the few remaining drips from his bottle and put it down next to the foot of his chair. He then lent forward and looked at me and said,

"If you knew 20 years ago what ICU medicine would be like today, do you think that you would still choose to be an intensivist?"

He paused, but not long enough for me to give an answer, and added,

"You know, I'm not so sure that I would."

John is about 10 to 15 years my junior. I last worked with him about 12 years ago when I knew him as a bright and enthusiastic intensivist who was a dedicated clinician, committed teacher and probing researcher. He continued with,

"Oh, I still get a kick every time I deal with a young critically ill patient who gets better and I still get a kick out of teaching, but I find that more and more of my time is being spent talking to relatives and taking them through the process of withdrawal of treatment for their dear old demented mother."

"Do you want another light beer?" I asked, and stood as if preparing for my errand.

"I've got stacks of it left in my fridge. My lads only leave the light beer as they reckon its poison," I added, trying to lighten the conversation.

John smiled a little but was not going to be moved.

"What do you think, Tub?" he repeated slowly "If you knew 20 years ago what ICU medicine would be like today, do you think that you would still choose to be an intensivist?"

I sat down again and began to peel the label from my bottle.

"Well . . . I know what you are saying and I guess that I am glad that I'm getting close to retirement, but I still think that I would."

We didn't continue the discussion much further. My wife had prepared the evening meal, the sun had set, and it was now becoming a little chilly so we went inside to eat. We spent the rest of the evening talking about other things. However, I could not forget our earlier conversation.

Intensive care is changing. I can remember when starting more than 35 years ago I worked in an 11-bedded intensive care unit which serviced a major teaching hospital with approximately 1000 beds (i.e. 1 ICU bed per 100 general hospital beds). We very rarely, if ever, admitted anyone over the age of 70. Withdrawal of therapy was an unusual event. The approach was simple, we treated patients actively until they survived or died.

Now, intensive care units vary from 20 - 40 beds in 400 - 800 bed hospitals (i.e. 1 ICU bed per 20 general hospital beds). The high dependency beds appear to have been incorporated into the ICU, patients are often more than 80 years old and intensivists are often required to withdraw therapy when there appears to be no hope of recovery. Withdrawal of therapy is now an important part of our practice.

I talked about this aspect of our vocation with two of our senior fellows, one of whom stated that during his training he had spent some time managing patients in a palliative care unit. He found, to his surprise, that palliation was a part of medicine that could be most rewarding, and that his time in that unit had prepared him well for this aspect of ICU medicine.

In the intensive care unit we do spend a lot of time talking to relatives. In the case of a frail elderly patient who is unconscious and unable to effectively communicate his or her wishes, where continued therapy is in question, we ask the relatives to articulate, as best they can, the patient's wishes after explaining to them the circumstances and likely prognosis. The discussions are involved, as there may be an almost limitless number of contingencies in which supportive therapy (e.g. cardiopulmonary resuscitation dialysis, ventilation, artificial feeding, life-sustaining drugs) may, or may not, be considered appropriate.

If withdrawal of therapy is considered desirable, the process is complex. It is not an abandonment of the patient or relatives. Perceptive management of both the patient's and relatives' physical and psychological needs throughout the ordeal, although at times delicate and demanding, is essential.

The ideal intensive care unit: open, closed or somewhere between?

"Poor is the pupil that does not surpass his master."
Leonardo Da Vinci

Some time ago a newly appointed junior surgeon to our hospital towered over the intensive care unit nursing chart and questioned the nurse about a recent order.

"Who ordered this for my patient?"

"Dr. Worthley did," she replied.

"Well, please tell him that I would like to see him!" he barked.

"He's in his room just down the hallway if you would like to see him" and moved to direct him.

"No I want him here now!"

The nurse hurried to my room and peeked around the door "Mr. Smith wants to see you about the new patient."

I smiled. "I heard the conversation from here," I said wearily as I stood, stretched and walked slowly to the ICU bed. I held my ire in check as I knew that this would probably be another typical exchange that not infrequently occurred during my earlier years as an intensivist.

"G'day you must be the new appointee to the Grant surgical unit. I remember discussing your curriculum vitae with the selection committee prior to your appointment. I wonder if we could talk in my office."

He looked a little perplexed at my introduction, possibly trying to assess my position in the political 'pecking order' within the hospital. He then straightened.

"I would prefer to discuss the patient here."

I bared my teeth; "Sure - but perhaps in my office first," I gestured to my door whilst walking away. He reluctantly followed, but slowly gained pace so as to reach my room first. As I entered I pulled the door shut, offered him a seat and brought my chair from behind the desk to allow me to face him directly.

Inside God's Shed

"Before we discuss the patient's treatment I think I should make the clinical responsibility of patients in our ICU quite clear. The primary responsibility for treatment is with the intensivist; we consult with the home team and other specialists when the need arises. We don't have 'his' or 'her' patients, we have 'our' patients and in the event that the home team feels that there may be aspects of our treatment that require explanation, we are only too happy to discuss this with them – civilly."

"You manage all the surgical problems then?" he scoffed.

"If we believe that there is an operative problem we will notify the home team of our concerns. However, when cardiac, respiratory, renal or infective problems develop, we will manage these without notifying the home team first: the same way that a surgeon who operates on a patient with an acute abdomen referred to him by a physician does not contact the physician during the operation to ask for permission or advice."

We continued our robust discussion, although I would add that following this episode 'Smithy' and I have become firm friends. He now respects the intensivist's opinion and while he initially threatened to stop sending all his acutely ill patients to the ICU, he now demands that they be admitted to our unit. Indeed, confrontation between a home clinic and the intensivist in relation to patient management is now rare and more often relates to bed unavailability.

Recently, I was amazed to learn that a new graduate intensivist preferred to work in an ICU that functioned more as an 'open' unit compared with ours, which prompted me to reconsider the concept of intensive care medicine as a specialty and the idea of 'open' and 'closed' units. A 'closed' unit – like ours – is defined as one where all care is directed by the resident intensivist. An 'open' unit is defined as one where the admitting clinician directs all treatment[1] or where an intensivist will be consulted only at the discretion of the admitting clinician.[2] The terms 'open' and 'closed' are not ideal descriptors. They tend to indicate a culture of inclusion for 'open' units and exclusion for 'closed' units, which is incorrect as it simply relates to who directs the patient's care. The terms 'service' units for open ICU's and

155

'specialist' units for closed ICU's may represent the operative status more precisely.

While Australasian ICU's generally function with the intensivist being primarily responsible for the patient's care (i.e. they manage critically ill patients in a 'closed' unit), the College of Intensive Care Medicine of Australia and New Zealand does not mention the words 'open' or 'closed' in their documents classifying Level I, II and III intensive care units. Nevertheless, with a common certification process, there is a broadly similar approach to patient care by the majority of Australasian intensivists,[3] and it would be the minority only who would embrace the concept of managing critically ill patients in an 'open' or service unit.

To work as an intensivist in an 'open' unit would require one to act largely as medical broker (i.e. one who has a broad smile, a long list of telephone numbers and who is without a contrary view), consulting widely for cardiac, respiratory, renal, etc opinions. However this tends to generate a range of conflicting options that causes confusion in the management of the critically ill patient. Indeed, there are many studies that have recorded an improvement in morbidity and mortality when critically ill patients are cared for in a 'closed' unit compared with those who are managed in an 'open' unit,[2,4,5,6,7,8,9,10,11] indicating at the very least that an 'open' model is not ideal.

As to the idea of a 'more open' unit (e.g. some of the ICU patients managed by the intensivist and the rest managed by the home team); it's a concept that's not commonly promoted by either 'open' or 'closed' unit advocates. It's like wanting to be half pregnant. However, if the intensivist in wanting to work in a 'more open' unit is expressing a wish to have less responsibility, this may indicate that his or her training is incomplete.

REFERENCES
1. Worthley LIG. Why do we continually ask "Do we need Intensivists"? Crit Care Resusc 2000;2:241-242.
2. Pronovost PJ, Angus DC, Dorman T, Robinson KA, Dremsizov TT, Young TL. Physician staffing patterns and clinical outcomes in

critically ill patients: a systematic review. JAMA 2002;288:2151-2162.
3. Worthley LIG. Peer review, standards, judgement and sweet charity. Crit Care Resusc 2003;5:309-310.
4. Brown JJ, Sullivan G. Effect on ICU mortality of a full time critical care specialist. Chest 1989;96:127-129.
5. Reynolds HN, Haupt MT, Thill-Baharozian MC, Carlson RW. Impact of critical care physician staffing on patients with septic shock in a university hospital medical intensive care unit. JAMA 1988;260:3446-3450.
6. Ghorra S, Reinert SE, Cioffi W, Buczko G, Simms HH. Analysis of the effect of conversion from open to closed surgical intensive care unit. Ann Surg 1999;229:163-171.
7. Carlson RW, Weiland DE, Strivasthan K. Does a full-time, 24 hour intensivist improve care and efficiency? Crit Care Clin 1996;12:525-551.
8. Hanson CW 3rd, Deutschman CS, Anderson HL 3rd, Reilly PM, Behringer EC, Schwab CW, et al. Effects of an organized critical care service on outcomes and resource utilization: a cohort study. Crit Care Med 1999;27:270-274.
9. Carson SS, Stocking C, Podsadecki T, Christenson J, Pohlman A, MacRae S, et al. Effects of organizational change in the medical intensive care unit of a teaching hospital. JAMA 1996;276:322-328.
10. Manthous CA, Amoateng-Adjepong Y, Al-Kharrat T, Jacob B, Alnuaimat HM, Chatila W, et al. Effects of a medical intensivist on patient care in a community teaching hospital. Mayo Clin Proc 1997;72:391-399.
11. Pronovost PJ, Jenckes MW, Dorman T, Garrett E, Breslow MJ, Rosenfeld BA, et al. Organizational characteristics of intensive care units related to outcomes of abdominal aortic surgery. JAMA 1999;281:1310-1317.

The pro – con debate: educational, or just another blood sport?

"Academic disputes are so bitter because the stakes are so small."
Henry Kissinger

Recently, I agreed to take part in a 'pro-con' debate regarding the Stewart approach to acid-base balance (i.e. 'Is the plasma pH regulated by strong ions?'). I took the 'con' position (i.e. the Stewart approach is flawed or 'Strong ion difference: a new paradigm or new clothes for the acid-base emperor?'). However I promptly found myself on the back foot when I learnt that one of my co-chairmen was a 'pro' supporter and had been embarrassed by me 24 hours ago when I, as his chairman, implied in front of a large audience that he had run over time. I waited for my invitation to the podium with some trepidation.

The pro side was advanced first, with the dialogue varying, along with various relevant points, from light humour to outright vilification of the con position. No problem, I have a reasonably robust ego – although it was telling me that I had not included enough 'clever' slides for my talk. I began, half expecting the time buzzer to be pushed ruthlessly and relentlessly. Unfortunately, as I proceeded I found that my Powerpoint® presentation had a font variance with the venue's computer, producing post-box and bifocal icons within important equations – confusing all as I tried to emphasise my point of view. Not a good start!

The right of reply involved a denigration of each other's position. However, my opponent had gone to more trouble than I, by using video 'bites' from various science fiction films that depicted me as a prince of darkness who was of questionable intellect. My response was less confronting. Should have I done more? Perhaps an incendiary sensory stimulus followed by an announcement that 'Elvis has now left the building'?

Nevertheless, the session went reasonably well and I was interested in the audience response. This ranged from a misunderstanding of the principles of hydrogen ion metabolism ("can someone explain why water with a pH of 7.0 at 25°C becomes more acidic when its temperature rises?") to an astute observation of the data presented ("In your slide listing the five equations, the fourth was wrong as it had a positive rather than negative superscript"), indicating that at least some were not distracted by the session's 'cut and thrust' approach, or my font variations.

After the meeting I wondered as to the educational value of the pro-con debate. Normally, techniques used to present medical data range from the 10-minute scientific report to the didactic lecture. In this regard, the pro-con debate is a relatively new educational tool, employing an adversarial structure where denigration of one position is used to support the validity of another. The presenters are generally unwilling to acknowledge any area of common ground and as the adversarial structure tends to promote the entertainment aspects of an argument, fidelity and precision of the evidence is often sidelined.

When discussing the topic informally with some of the registrants after the session, I found no swinging voters (i.e. those who had changed their mind after the event). The session appeared to polarise the audience, strengthening preconceived ideas and prejudices, rather than promoting an analysis or evaluation of facts.

Science (if that is what Medicine is), unlike art (unless that is what Medicine is), does not boast an eternal truth. With constant questioning and experimentation, facts and theories change. With this in mind, one should teach the student to think critically, to question paradigms and to challenge all past, present, and future models with an open mind.

Nevertheless, it is not just knowledge or understanding that one wishes to impart, it's curiosity, enthusiasm, scepticism, excitement and passion. Education is not filling a bucket, but lighting a fire and humour is often used to achieve this. However, the teacher is not just an entertainer and the humour used to facilitate learning is probably not that of derision.

Intravenous albumin: a waste of health dollars?

"There are some remedies worse than the disease."
Publilius Syrus

Some time ago I was asked to speak at a local meeting of the Australasian Association of Clinical Biochemists. The title of my presentation, *'Intravenous albumin: a waste of health dollars?'*, I thought was probably provocative enough for the local biochemists, as I knew most of them well and enjoyed their company. However, when I arrived and was told that it was a Joint Teleconference with the Victorian Branch of the Australasian Association of Clinical Biochemists, I wasn't so sure they would be quite as tolerant of my presentation as the local group.

Nevertheless, I began with the fundamental features of albumin, explaining that albumin is a protein that appeared early in evolution, and in humans is a single polypeptide containing 585 amino acids. It has a molecular weight of 66248 and is responsible for approximately 70% of the plasma oncotic pressure (i.e. the osmotic pressure caused by plasma proteins). The total body albumin is 4 - 5 g/kg body weight (i.e. approximately 350 g in an adult human), 40% of which resides in the intravascular space (in blood) and 60% resides in the interstitial space (i.e. the space external to body cells and blood).[1]

As nobody demurred with my introductory statements, I continued by saying that normal albumin production, in the adult human, ranges from 10 - 25 g/day[1] and can increase to a maximum of approximately 50 g/day.[2] It has a half-life of 20 days[3] and its production is largely regulated by the hepatic interstitial oncotic pressure.[4] It transports free fatty acids, bilirubin, hormones (e.g. thyroxine, cortisol), binds calcium, copper and mercury ions and many drugs, and can scavenge oxygen free radicals.[2,5] Albumin also has anticoagulant activities and is responsible for maintaining normal capillary permeability to protein.[5]

Inside God's Shed

Both the South Australian and Victorian tele-audience were either happy with what I had said so far or were nodding off. However, I thought that my next few comments would stimulate some reaction, so I continued.

"Albumin synthesis is increased by increasing insulin, thyroxine and cortisol levels[6] and decreased by the inflammatory cytokines, TNF-α and IL-6.[7] Serum albumin levels are regulated by its production, degradation (or loss) and capillary permeability (varying the blood to interstitial compartment ratio).[8,9] However the reduction in albumin production, due to inflammatory cytokines,[7,10,11] and increased albumin transfer from blood to the interstitial space (due to an increase in capillary permeability) [12,13,14,15] with critical illness, is a normal response to inflammation."

"Ladies and gentlemen," I explained, "hypoalbuminaemia in the critically ill, is a indicator of the severity of illness, it is not a disease."

I had only delivered the first 10 minutes of my 40 minute talk, and could see that the local biochemists were beginning to smile, and on the video screen the Victorian Group were becoming restless. "Good," I thought, and continued to develop my proposition that *albumin therapy was a waste of health dollars*.

I stated that there are a group of individuals who have been born with a rare congenital absence or extremely low levels of serum albumin. This condition is known as analbuminaemia. These individuals are often asymptomatic or demonstrate only mild peripheral oedema,[16,17] and in spite of high cholesterol values and high levels of plasma clotting factors they may live a normal life span in the absence of atherosclerosis or thrombotic events.[18]

"Ladies and gentlemen," I pronounced, "hypoalbuminaemia is not lethal!"

"Ahh, but that's chronic hypoalbuminaemia, where an increase in α1, α2 and β globulins compensate for the reduction in albumin. Acute hypoalbuminaemia does not have this effect and has been known for years to be associated with an increased mortality," a shrill voice from the television console proclaimed.

Unfortunately, the visual display of the tele-audience followed the sound by a few seconds and was a little distracting. Nevertheless, the Victorian biochemist behind the voice soon came into view.

"That's absolutely true," I said, "and patients who have terminal cancer have a high incidence of having a nose. Just because there is an association between two things does not mean that one causes the other," I said to a screen that was showing images that varied between being frozen and animated.

"That argument is ludicrous!" he responded. "Severe malnutrition is well known to cause low albumin levels and high mortality."

The local biochemists presumably knew that the Victorian group were a little feisty and started to chuckle.

"Well," I added, "concerning malnutrition, while patients with kwashiorkor (i.e. malnutrition due to a reduced intake of protein without a similar reduction in carbohydrate) have severe hypoalbuminaemia, patients who have marasmus (i.e. malnutrition due to a reduced intake of carbohydrate, fat and protein) often have normal plasma albumin levels.[19] Albumin levels are not a sensitive or specific marker of malnutrition, and should not be used as a nutritional marker in humans.[20] Furthermore," I added, "there have been no studies to date that have shown intravenous albumin to treat hypoalbuminaemia, whatever its cause, reduces mortality."

"So acute hypoalbuminaemia doesn't trouble you then?" said the Victorian biochemist who appeared intermittently on the televised screen.

I realized at this point I was having an interactive session with the Victorian group only. The South Australian audience were simply onlookers – perhaps voyeurs?

"No," I replied and continued, "albumin solutions have been used to correct hypoalbuminaemia in the belief that they will reduce the incidence of pulmonary oedema, gastrointestinal oedema, peripheral oedema and mortality.[21] In the only randomized controlled studies to date of critically ill patients with albumin levels less than 25 g/L, albumin infusions did not reduce the complication rate, length of hospital stay or mortality rate.[22,23] In brief," I concluded, "giving patients intravenous albumin is useless!"

Inside God's Shed

"So is there no blood level of albumin that worries you then? What about 15 g/L, or 10 g/L, what about 5 g/L?" The Victorian biochemist obviously believed that there was a point at which I would have to acquiesce. I could see the image of the Victorian group motionless and in clear focus. "When would you administer albumin?" the Victorian biochemist boomed.

"Even at nought, donut, zip or zero grams per litre, I would not give intravenous albumin. Hypoalbuminaemia is not a disease," I fired back.

The next image of the Victorian group was one of an uproar – laughing, cheering and applauding. They understood my message, and as a veteran intensivist they were probably willing to believe me.

We live in a measurement-obsessed community in an imperfect world. What is valuable gets measured and what gets measured is given value. The intensivist often has to deal daily with an enormous array of numbers generated from various instruments. The numbers are compared with those values that are found in 95% of normal individuals who are supine, at rest, and have been fasting, and, by implication, values that lie outside this 'normal' range must be acted upon. However, values that lie outside the 'normal' range should be reviewed in the context of the underlying disease. Numbers are symbols that should be carefully interpreted. If they represent an abnormality caused by disease, the disease should be treated. Twiddling a number by itself is not necessarily associated with a better outcome, and not understanding the physiological or pathophysiological processes involved is a poor platform upon which to base therapy.

Giving intravenous albumin to hypoalbuminaemic patients treats a number; it does not cure a disease.

Postscript.
I presented the lecture *"Intravenous albumin: a waste of health dollars?"* in 1998. In 1999 a prospective randomised, multicentre, controlled trial in patients who had cirrhosis with ascites and spontaneous bacterial peritonitis, a reduction in renal impairment (from 33% to 10%) and in hospital mortality (from 29% to 10%) and three month

mortality (from 41% to 22%) using intravenous albumin (1.5 g/kg bodyweight within 6 hours of detecting the infection and 1 g/kg on day three) was reported.[24] However, this study was flawed as it was not blinded and the control group received inadequate fluid therapy.[25]

In 2011, a Cochrane collaboration study concluded that "for patients with hypovolaemia, there is no evidence that albumin reduces mortality when compared with cheaper alternatives such as saline", adding that "there is no evidence that albumin reduces mortality in critically ill patients with burns and hypoalbuminaemia".[26]

REFERENCES
1. Doweiko JP, Nompleggi DJ. Role of albumin in human physiology and pathophysiology. J Parenter Enteral Nutr 1991;15:207-211.
2. Rothschild MA, Oratz M, Schreiber SS. Serum albumin. Hepatology 1988;8:385-401
3. Klein S. The myth of serum albumin as a measure of nutritional status. Gastroenterology 1990;99:1845-1846.
4. Pietrangelo A, Panduro A, Chowdhury JR, Shafritz DA Albumin gene expression is down-regulated by albumin or macromolecule infusion in the rat. J Clin Invest 1992;89:1755-1760.
5. Emerson TE Jr. Unique features of albumin: a brief review. Crit Care Med 1989;17:690-694.
6. Kimball SR, Horetsky RL, Jefferson LS Hormonal regulation of albumin gene expression in primary cultures of rat hepatocytes. Am J Physiol 1995;268:E6-E14.
7. Nicholson JP, Wolmarans MR, Park GR. The role of albumin in critical illness. Br J Anaesth 2000;85:599-610.
8. Rothschild MA, Oratz M, Schreiber SS. Albumin synthesis (First of two parts). N Engl J Med 1972;286:748-757.
9. Rothschild MA, Oratz M, Schreiber SS. Albumin synthesis (Second of two parts). N Engl J Med 1972;286:816-821.
10. Klein S. The myth of serum albumin as a measure of nutritional status. Gastroenterology 1990;99:1845-1846.
11. Soeters PB, von Meyenfeldt MF, Meijerink WJ, Fredrix EW, Wouters EFM, Schols AM. Serum albumin and mortality. Lancet 1990;335(8685):348.

12. Courtney ME, Greene HL, Folk CC, Helinek GL, Dmitruk A. Rapidly declining serum albumin values in newly hospitalized patients: prevalence, severity, and contributory factors. J Parenter Enteral Nutr 1982;6:143-145.
13. Fleck A. Raines G, Hawker F, Trotter J, Wallace PI, Ledingham I McA, et al. Increased vascular permeability: a major cause of hypoalbuminaemia in disease and injury. Lancet 1985;1(8432):781-784.
14. O'Keefe SJD, Dicker J. Is the plasma albumin concentration useful in the assessment of nutritional status of hospital patients? Eur J Clin Nutr 1988;42:41-45.
15. Boosalis MG, Ott L, Levine AS, Slag MF, Morley JE, Young B, et al. Relationship of visceral proteins to nutritional status in chronic and acute stress. Crit Care Med 1989;17:741-747.
16. Russi E, Weigand K. Analbuminemia. Klin Wochenschr 1983;61:541-545.
17. Dammacco F, Miglietta A, D'Addabbo A, Fratello A, Moschetta R, Bonomo L. Analbuminemia: report of a case and review of the literature. Vox Sang 1980;39:153-161.
18. Kallee E. Bennhold's analbuminemia: a follow-up study of the first two cases (1953-1992). J Lab Clin Med 1996;127:470-480.
19. McLaren DS. A fresh look at protein-energy malnutrition in the hospitalized patient. Nutrition 1988;4:1-6.
20. Jeejeebhoy KN. Nutrition and serum albumin levels. Nutrition 1994;10:353.
21. Kaminski MV, Williams SD. Review of the rapid normalization of serum albumin with mofdified total parenteral nutrition solutions. Crit Care Med 1990;18:327-335.
22. Foley EF, Borlase BC, Dzik WH, Bistrian BR, Benotti PN. Albumin supplementation in the critically ill. A prospective, randomized trial. Arch Surg 1990;125:739-742.
23. Rubin H, Carlson S, DeMeo M, Granger D, Craig RM. Randomized, double-blind study of intravenous human albumin in hypoalbuminemic patients receiving total parenteral nutrition. Crit Care med 1997;25:249-252.

24. Sort P, Navasa M, Arroyo V, Aldeguer X, Planas R, Ruiz-del-Arbol L, et al. Effect of intravenous albumin on renal impairment and mortality in patients with cirrhosis and spontaneous bacterial peritonitis. N Engl J Med 1999;341:403-409.
25. Patch D, Burroughs A. Intravenous albumin in patients with cirrhosis and spontaneous bacterial peritonitis. N Engl J Med 1999;341:1773-1774.
26. Roberts I, Blackhall K, Anderson P, Bunn F, Schierhout G. Human albumin solution for resuscitation and volume expansion in critically ill patients. Cochrane Database Syst Rev 2011 Nov 9;11:CD001208.

Naked in the electronic age

"I like to do all the talking myself. It saves time, and prevents arguments."
Oscar Wilde

I received an invitation a few months ago to hear a talk from a visiting speaker about 'current management of venous thromboembolism' and I immediately did a 'PubMed' (www.ncbi.nlm.nih.gov/pubmed) Medline search on the speaker's publications. Not only was the individual's list of publications short, but also none were written on the topic he was invited to discuss.

I had just stripped the speaker bare, and was about to throw my invitation into the waste basket when I began wondering just how well would I fare under the same scrutiny. I've been asked as a visiting speaker to present a topic that I've not published on. After the presentation the audience seemed to be happy – were they just courteous? Perhaps there were many invitations to my presentation that hit the bottom of the bin – who knows.

Just then one of my work-mates passed my door so I said "Andrew, do you 'PubMed' speakers before you go to their talk?"

"Yes" was the reply as he stepped back to the doorway.

"Well what do you do if their CV's are a bit thin?"

He paused and frowned a little and looked past me as if reading something on the wall written in very small letters. "Well, sometimes I go and sometimes I don't. If the speaker has a reputation of being interesting – I might go."

"Gee, 'PubMed' me and I don't look all that good," I said.

Andrew grinned and turned, "All your talks go to the bin, mate," he replied, and left.

I knew that he was half joking, but it was the other half that left me a bit bothered. Generally, I felt that when I gave a talk I knew how my presentations had been received, by the applause. Loud and prolonged – good; light and short – OK. Sometimes there is a gentle polite acclamation followed by an uncomfortable silence during question time, with the chairman desperately attempting to think of a relevant question to begin the discussion – probably bad. If there is just silence – very bad.

I began thinking about the features I found necessary during my presentations to ensure that my message, if not remembered, was at least thought provoking. It appeared to me that it largely required time and skill. Mark Twain said, "it usually takes me more than three weeks to prepare a good impromptu speech". Concerning skill, Winston Churchill said that when delivering a speech "it should have a strong beginning, focus on one theme, use simple language, draw a picture in the listener's mind, and end with an emotion."

One of the major criticisms of the modern medical presentation is that it has become 'far too serious' and that the object of the clinician should be to 'entertain and educate in that order'.[1] To educate, the medical speaker should be experienced and informed.[2] Experience, for better or worse, comes with age. To become informed, one has to research and publish, and I guess that is where the 'PubMed' search is of value.

However, to be an entertaining speaker requires not just a joke at the beginning and one at the end, it requires a performance. It should be stylish, even flamboyant, with a variation in voice tone and a delivery implying a sense of fun. The lecture should not be read, nor should it be memorised word for word. The former leads to a monotonous tone from a head buried in the lectern, and the latter tends to lead to a complex dissertation of the written word, rather than a clear and simple message given in the spoken word. The important points of a talk should be remembered and used as stepping stones; one may even 'ride on a set of slides' or, at worst, use prompt cards.

It seems to me that the essential elements for one wishing to present a thought provoking and memorable message are:
- know your subject. Have your presentation organised (e.g. Introduction: why did we do it? Methods: what did we do? Results: what did we find? Discussion and Conclusion: what does it all mean?)
- catch the attention of your audience. Be provocative. For example, when talking about pain relief in the intensive care

patient, speak to a title such as 'pain never killed anybody, but pain relief has'.
- impart a sense of enthusiasm, curiosity, scepticism, excitement, and passion for your work.
- speak deliberately (almost slowly). Speak clearly, 'carve every word before you let it fall'. Add light and shade to the tone of your voice. By inflection you can say much more than your words do.
- humour. Don't take yourself too seriously (although don't clown, as you do want others to take you seriously).
- be confident. Look momentarily at each visible face in the audience.
- design visual aids (e.g. slides) simply (e.g. horizontal format, no more than 5 to 7 lines per slide and 3 to 6 words per line with a space of at least the height of a letter between lines)[3] and legibly.[4]
- on average use one slide per minute.[5] Do not go over-board with the visual or audio features of PowerPoint®.
- at question time, have a sense of humility (not timidity) be humble (not weak) and acknowledge other workers in your field and people who have helped you.
- finally, and most importantly, practice your talk, preferably in front of your peers.[6] DO NOT GO OVERTIME. Your 10-minute talk should last for 9 minutes.[7] Your 30-minute talk should last for 20 minutes, and the 60-minute talk 45 minutes.

Apart from gauging the response to your talk by the applause at the end, if the presentation has been fun it is likely that you have also provided a very enjoyable talk for your audience.

REFERENCES
1. Calnan J. Medical research, reading, speaking and writing. Proc R Soc Med 1977;70:454-455.
2. Calnan J. A lecture on lecturing. Med Educ 1976;10:445-449.

3. Garson A Jr, Gutgesell HP, Pinsky WW, McNamara DG. The 10 minute talk: organization, slides, writing, and delivery. Am Heart J 1986;111:193-203.
4. Battle JD Jr. Selected for presentation. Arch Intern Med 1978;138:1697.
5. Kroenke K. The 10-minute talk. Am J Med 1987;83:329-330.
6. Cull P. Making and using medical slides. Br J Hosp Med 1992;47:132-135.
7. Garson A Jr. Meeting improvement: a guide to preparation of "slides" for presentation. J Am Coll Cardiol 1999;34:886-889.

"We have a unique opportunity to offer you the newest treatment for...."

"It takes a disciplined person to listen to convictions which are different from their own."
Dorothy Fuldheim

There is little doubt that many of the major therapeutic advances in medicine have been initiated by medical research. Experimental drugs designed from basic research and tested in experimental models may indicate potential benefits of these new agents. However, it's human research, which depends upon large prospective randomized controlled trials, that provides real evidence of clinical benefit, or otherwise, of the new drug. Moreover, before a doctor begins to have confidence in any new therapy, research must be able to be confirmed by others, eliminating any hidden or overt bias that may have existed in the original study.

Research in patients with a disease for which new drugs are thought to be of benefit, requires informed consent. If the patient is to give consent to be enrolled in a trial, he or she must be informed of: the current standard treatment for the illness, the probability of a beneficial outcome and what the benefit(s) and side-effects of standard treatment are and how these may compare with the 'new' therapy. The trial must also have approval from the institution's ethics committee.

To be truly informed, the patient may find it a little disconcerting to be told; "We do not know the best way to treat your condition when comparing the 'standard' treatment with our proposed new treatment, as the new treatment may be; better, not be worse or be worse than standard treatment. And the treatment you receive will be determined by the toss of a coin."

It is usually anticipated by the researchers that the differences between treatments may be large, as they often have a preconceived belief as to the beneficial effect of the new therapy. There are often vested interests as well (to promote status, position, advancement and funding) that help drive the enrolment of patients. Accordingly, the statement "we do not know the best way...." rarely prefixes the conversation between the researcher and patient. To enhance the enrolment of patients the dialogue tends be more 'promotional'.

I was asked to review a patient in a general ward who had chronic respiratory failure and overheard a doctor in the next bay talking to a patient who had been admitted with a diagnosis of an acute coronary syndrome. The patient still had chest pain. He had just been admitted from the A&E department where a doctor told him he had a critical reduction in the blood supply to his heart and that he needed an urgent procedure to widen the offending vessel. The diagnosis and the curative treatment appeared to be clear in the patient's mind. However in the ward, his doctor, who had just finished his clinical examination, argued against the A&E doctor's advice and said that he may not benefit from the intervention as much as that which could be achieved using a new therapeutic approach to his condition.

"We have a unique opportunity to offer you the newest treatment for your heart disease. It will thin your blood as well as reduce the activity of your heart to stabilize your condition and reduce the chance of you having an adverse outcome associated with the percutaneous procedure that is planned for you."

"Really," I thought.

I knew the research fellow who would have prompted the resident doctor attempting to gain informed consent for his study. I had listened to him recently give a talk about the newer anticoagulant drugs and autonomic system blockers in patients who have had an acute coronary syndrome. It was exciting to hear someone who had such a passion for his work. However there was a patient at the end of this 'informed consent' procedure, enduring a spiel that sounded more like an advertising campaign than a prelude to informed consent.

The patient was then asked to consider the study for a few moments while the doctor left to get some papers for him to sign, adding that whether he received the standard or newer treatment would be determined at random.

The patient, I am sure, was confused. If he agreed to be enrolled in the study, his percutaneous procedure – he probably could envisage this 'curing' his blocked coronary artery – or 'newer' drug therapy – he probably did not have the same confidence as the researcher in this curing his disease – would be chosen at random. Moreover, if he refused to be enrolled in the study, would his doctor still have the same interest in managing him?

There are many conflicts of interest in medical research. One may even have a grant that depends upon the department enrolling a certain number of patients.

While the researcher, I'm sure, genuinely believed that he could offer the patient a better treatment than the standard therapy, informed consent is vital in the process of research. The conversation between a researcher and patient has to be honest, with the understanding that there will be no positive or negative influences imposed on the patient if they decline to be enrolled. The doctor undertaking informed consent should be completely detached from the research project and taught by the institution's ethics committee as to the appropriate conversation when gaining consent, even if recruitment to a trial may be prejudiced.

Clinicians must act in the best interests of the patient under their care. If they betray this commitment, even for a cause that may benefit future patients, the doctor–patient relationship is violated.[1]

REFERENCES
1. Angell M. Patients' preferences in randomized clinical trials. N Engl J Med 1984;310:1385-1387.

The scientific journal: editorial freedom, freedom of expression and the pursuit of truth

"You know the old adage, 'If it sounds too good to be true, it probably is'? Conversely, If it sounds too bad to be true, it also probably is!"
Betsy Crowfoot

A scientific journal publishes research that has undergone an exacting and impartial review from 3 to 4 expert reviewers. It's a process known as peer review. It ensures that research is accepted and published only when the study meets a certain standard, the findings are sound and the conclusions valid. The journal should also have a conflict of interest policy and a correspondence section. The latter allows for free, perceptive and robust discussion of the author's findings by the wider scientific community and is an important part of the review process. Editorial independence, impartiality, integrity and transparency are fundamental tenets of the scientific journal and should not be subject to the discretion of any organization.

To meet the objectives of an independent and impartial review requires a scientific community that is committed to the pursuit of truth without prejudice. However this is often difficult to achieve, as a reviewer will tend to have personal beliefs and vested interests in the subject being reviewed. This means that a totally detached process is practically impossible, as a completely unbiased scientist is unlikely to be an expert on the subject under review. For example, the reviewers may be preoccupied with their own position and status and are reviewing the work of competitors for funds. They may even be bitter rivals. Nevertheless, the peer review process is probably the most effective way of exercising quality control of the work presented, and chief editors have an important role to play in assessing any reviewer bias.

However the chief editor of the journal must be free from any organizational prerogative. At a meeting of the International Committee of Medical Journal Editors, a statement supporting editorial freedom in relation to medical journals was prepared and promulgated.[1] While this may appear to be a 'given' for any publication purporting to advance academic activities, there are examples in the medical realm where this freedom may be qualified. The dismissal of George Lundberg, some time ago, as the editor-in-chief of the Journal of the American Medical Association (JAMA) by the executive of the American Medical Association, prompted the editor of the Lancet to state that 'JAMA is no longer part of a free press'.[2] The events that led to the dismissal of the editor-in-chief involved a JAMA press release commenting about an article on what type of activity a cohort of college students believed having 'sex' meant. The press release stated that the 'issue is of particular interest and debate now because of recent presidential statements'.

The reason for the dismissal? Apparently George Lundberg had 'threatened the historic tradition and integrity of JAMA by inappropriately and inexcusably interjecting into a major political debate that has nothing to do with science or medicine'. In a prophetic twist, in 1988 when George Lundberg wrote an editorial in the JAMA discussing editorial freedom, he quoted Hugh Clegg (Quondam Editor, British Medical Journal) as saying, "a medical editor has to be a keeper of the conscience of a profession; if he tries to live up to this ideal he will always be getting into trouble."[3]

To meet the objectives of integrity and transparency, the journal must be free from political activists and advocacy. Advocacy science tends to blur the distinction between science informing political leaders about policy and science directing policy. Winston Churchill believed that "experts should always be on tap and never on top". Scientific journals should report facts and be cautious about being drawn into offering a polemic. Whenever science acquires the role of directly authorising policy it tends to encourage a paternalistic political administration that claim a privileged access to a higher cause. In this regard the Intergovernmental Panel on Climate Change (IPCC) came under intense criticism with its early reports. For example, a review of the statement that the 'IPCC Fourth Assessment Report *Climate Change 2007* based their recommendations only on peer reviewed studies', found that of the 18,531 references cited in the report, 5,587 (30%) were from non-peer reviewed articles.[4] Moreover, experts had been chosen for geographical and gender balance rather than their expertise and knowledge. These problems of integrity do not enhance the reputation of scientists and the scientific process. Truth becomes a casualty.

Concerning medical science: In his Pulitzer prize winning book 'The Emperor of all Maladies', Siddhartha Mukherjee outlined the chronology of one attempt to push forward what was genuinely believed at the time to be ground-breaking science in the treatment of breast cancer. In 1999, Dr. Bezwoda, a breast cancer researcher from South Africa, presented a paper showing remarkably successful results with high-dose chemotherapy followed by bone marrow transplantation (BMT) in breast cancer patients.[5] In a "liberating moment for many patients and patient advocates", seven American state legislatures enacted laws requiring health maintenance organisations to pay for high dose chemotherapy and BMT for patients with advanced breast cancer. Similar legislation pended in seven more states.[6] However, other clinicians could not reproduce Dr. Bezwoda's results. Subsequently, a team of investigators visited his unit to explore his methods, only to find misleading data. He finally admitted to outright fraud, and in a public statement wrote, "I hereby acknowledge that I have committed a serious breach of scientific honesty and integrity."[7] When the truth finally emerged from subsequent trials in patients with advanced breast cancer treated with high dose chemotherapy and BMT, no benefit could be found.[8]

To the scientific mind eternal truth is a myth. Words such as 'incontrovertible' are an anathema.[9] The true scientific mind constantly questions. By definition a scientist is a sceptic. What is not widely understood by the public is that in science you cannot know with certainty a proposition is true; you can only know that it was not true.[10] Einstein knew this by stating "no amount of experimentation can ever prove me right; a single experiment can prove me wrong."

Science can only be created by those who are driven toward truth and understanding. Not by those who are driven by ideas of good and bad.

REFERENCES
1. Editorial freedom: A Statement by the International Committee of Medical Journal Editors. Lancet 1988;2(8619):1089.
2. Horton R. The sacking of JAMA. Lancet 1999;353(9149):252-253.
3. Lundberg GD. Editorial freedom and integrity. JAMA 1988;260:2563.
4. Laframboise D. The delinquent teenager who was mistaken for the world's top climate expert. Toronto: Ivy Avenue Press, 2011.
5. Bezwoda WR. High dose chemotherapy with haematopoietic rescue in breast cancer. Hematol Cell Ther 1999;41:58-65.
6. Mukherjee S. The emperor of all maladies. New York: Schribner, 2010. P325.
7. Mukherjee S. The emperor of all maladies. New York: Schribner, 2010. P327-328.
8. Mukherjee S. The emperor of all maladies. New York: Schribner, 2010. P328.
9. Allegre C, Armstrong JS, Breslow J, Cohen R, David E, Happer W, et al. Climate change 'heretics' rebuff carbon dangers. The Australian, February 1, 2012 p14
10. Popper KR. The logic of scientific discovery. New York 1959.

"But . . . ?"

"Free inquiry requires that we tolerate diversity of opinion and that we respect the right of individuals to express their beliefs, however unpopular they may be, without social or legal prohibition or fear of success."
    Paul Kurtz

"I would like to congratulate the authors on their presentation - *but...*" is the commonly used platform following a scientific presentation from which any comment or question may be launched. While the prelude to the word 'but' may be taken by the speaker as a euphemism for disagreement, it should always be taken positively. In any educational forum, questioning is mandatory.

To the scientist everlasting truth is an illusion. It is the ability to ask the correct questions that deepens our knowledge, not the answers, as they will never be absolute. Karl Popper believed that "Science does not rest on solid bedrock. The bold structure of its theories arise, as it were, above a swamp. It is like a building erected on piles. The piles are driven down from above into the swamp, but not down to any natural or given base; and if we stop driving the piles deeper, it is not because we have reached firm ground. We simply stop when we are satisfied that the piles are firm enough to carry the structure, at least for the time being."[1]

To learn about a problem, facts and concepts must be probed continually, and in this context 'but' is a vital word. While, the preamble (and the word 'but') should be meant and taken with charity, occasionally it is an introduction to a question or a comment that may reveal more about the questioner than the topic under discussion. A good chairman is useful to redirect the focus in such circumstances.

As well as in the open scientific forum, in any scientific institution, the head of a department should foster constant questioning and encourage the alternate points of view. Even if this requires a robust review of his or her own 'pet' theories. The active and vibrant departments always seem to have individuals who lead with sincerity, enthusiasm and humility, describing their colleagues as 'wizards', always talking about 'we' and usually considering their own input into the various studies underway in their own departments as minor.

Nonetheless, there are caveats. While the future may belong to the skeptic, it does not belong to the cynic. Skepticism pursues evidence and is built on a genuine honesty for precision and fidelity; cynicism reflects more an arrogance of ignorance and seeks to destroy the virtue of any wish to seek the truth. Moreover, while Max Perutz (the discoverer of the structure of haemoglobin) may believe that "In science you don't have to be polite, you only have to be right", questioning with charity, courtesy and good will, allows the necessary questions to be asked without anyone losing face.

At all stages, different points of view must be encouraged. New attitudes and opinions foster creativity, initiative and, particularly relevant in our era, change. In this sense, problem finding or creative observation should be rewarded if not with an encouraging comment from our senior people, at least with a friendly smile. Learning and seeking truth is not a subversive activity, it only occurs when there is freedom of thought, ideas and expression.

REFERENCES
1. Popper KR. The logic of scientific discovery. London: Hutchinson and Co, 1959.

Section 4. Drug companies

Can a doctor enjoy a medical company's generosity without prescribing its products?

"*I fear Greeks even when they bring gifts.*"
   Virgil

"Would you rather me prescribe a drug to you or one of your family that I thought would work or would you rather my prescribing habits be influenced simply by drug promotion?" I said to the 'rep' who persisted in trying to get me to prescribe one of his company's 'wonder' drugs that had been recently included in the pharmaceutical benefits scheme.

"Well, if I am critically ill with severe sepsis, I hope that you would use our drug," the 'rep' responded.

Touché, I thought, use an emotional argument and you will get an emotional response.

The relationship between the medical profession and industry (i.e. pharmaceutical and instrument manufacturers and distributors) is an interesting one. Informally, we receive their representatives at our office with indifference. We banter with them at the trade display, give the trinkets they have on offer to our children (or grandchildren) and plead with them when we want financial support for research, travel or sponsoring for our scientific meetings. Nevertheless, within the formal relationship there is a code of conduct. For example, it is unethical to accept remuneration for participating in advertising or promotion of products. On the other hand, it is acceptable to provide services that include *bona fide* consultation and legal testimony, as well as institutionally approved product testing, evaluation and development by way of experimental and clinical research.

Inside God's Shed

While some companies appear to give money with 'no strings attached', medical corporations are no more altruistic with shareholders equity than any other business. No company gives away its shareholder's money in an act of disinterested generosity, so arrangements with the medical profession will only be entered into if they enhance the company's market share. However, some of these agreements (e.g. direct research grants, ownership of equity or options thereon and patent royalties) raise issues of conflict of interest and bias.

Bias induced by conflict of interest works subtly and is not the same as dishonest behaviour, which is why the double blind randomised controlled trial is so crucial to the scientific test. The International Committee of Medical Journal Editors defines conflict of interest, when an individual (e.g. author, reviewer, editor) has financial or personal relationships with other persons or organisations that inappropriately influence (i.e. bias) his or her actions.[1,2]

There are several instances in which medical industry funding may have influenced the conclusions of published articles.[3,4] In an epidemiological study of randomised clinical trials published in the British Medical Journal (BMJ) from January 1997 to June 2001, the authors conclusions significantly favoured the experimental interventions when financial competing interests (i.e. funding by for-profit organisations) were present, whereas other competing interests (e.g. personal, academic or political) did not appear to influence the authors conclusions.[5]

Nevertheless, to attempt to abolish all conflict of interest is impossible, and one may argue that the only person who does not have some sort of vested interest in a subject is somebody who knows nothing about it.[6] The BMJ's policy concerning conflict of interest is that it should be disclosed but not prohibited. Disclosure will allow the reader to consider this along with many other factors when making his or her judgment on the value of a study or report.[7] Editors of other journals, have also established policies to ensure that the financial associations of authors are disclosed.[8,9,10,11,12,13,14,15,16,17]

From an industry point of view, there is a belief that markets work on the principle that a product brings benefit to the user. If the

181

product is not beneficial, there is no market, or if the product is harmful the market will respond adversely, so it is not in the interests of a company to publish false facts or promote a useless (or harmful) product. Yet I wonder whether this reflects the truth. The tobacco industry highlights some of the activities that will occur, particularly when a CEO of a company is encouraged to focus on short-term market gains. Currently, there are whole university medical school departments that operate as subsidiaries of pharmaceutical companies.[18] They dictate terms of the trial, which may not necessarily be in the best interests of study participants or the advancement of science, and data may not be able to be examined independently.[19] In an attempt to gain a positive result, trials may use inappropriate controls (e.g. a dosing of two drugs that favours the experimental drug compared with the control drug[20]) or choose a narrow population base and extrapolate the conclusions inappropriately to a broader population affected by the condition.[21,22] Moreover, ghost-writing of entire medical research articles is now not uncommon.[23,24] Third party agencies, funded wholly by drug and device manufacturers, form partnerships with investigators to ensure that manuscripts submitted for publication have the proper spin. Information for physicians is carefully orchestrated with more than 100 for-profit medical communication companies to choose from.[25] So long as a drug does no harm, if it has promising experimental and clinical data and a pathophysiological mechanism that sounds reasonable, the rest may simply become a marketing exercise to hawk the product.

The selling of products through the use of not-for-profit organisation names and logos in advertising is a new trend. The industry understands that consumers place a high level of trust in non-profit organisations, believing that products that carry an endorsement by the non-profit organisation are superior to other competing products. In Australia we are beginning to see these effects. I was interested to read the title 'View from ANZICS' (the Australian and New Zealand Intensive Care Society) in a drug company publication reporting the use of drotrecogin alfa (Xigris® - Intensive Care News; issue 1: October 2002). A closer look revealed that the title simply alerted the reader to a column that a professor of intensive care would provide in future issues concerning updates 'on the intensive care world'. It was unclear if his title (President of the Australian and New Zealand Intensive Care Society) would be of any relevance to his presentation. For example, was it a view of, or report on, ANZICS activities (which are provided in the society's newsletter 'The Intensivist') or was it more significant for the title of the society (ANZICS) to be associated with the drug company's publication and therefore promotion of its products?

The many and varied influences to a practitioner's prescribing habits should be based on unbiased and sound scientific evidence. To the question: "can a doctor enjoy a company's generosity without prescribing its products?" - well for the patient's sake I certainly hope so.

REFERENCES
1. Conflict of interest. International Committee of Medical Journal Writers. Lancet 1993;341(8847):742-743.
2. Davidoff F, DeAngelis CD, Drazen JM, et al. Sponsorship, authorship, and accountability. Lancet 2001;358(9285):854-856.
3. Bodenheimer T. Uneasy alliance: clinical investigators and the pharmaceutical industry. N Engl J Med 2000;342:1539-1544.
4. Thomas PS, Tan KS, Yates DH. Sponsorship, authorship, and accountability. Lancet 2002;359(9303):351.
5. Kjaergard LL, Als-Nielsen B. Association between competing interests and authors' conclusions: epidemiological study of randomised clinical trials published in the BMJ. BMJ 2002;325:249-252.
6. Choudhry NK, Stelfox HT, Detsky AS. Relationships between authors of clinical practice guidelines and the pharmaceutical industry. JAMA 2002; 287: 612-617.
7. Smith R. Beyond conflict of interest. Transparency is the key. BMJ 1998;317:291-292.
8. Relman AS. Dealing with conflicts of interest. N Engl J Med 1984;310:1182-1183.
9. Rennie D, Flanagin A, Glass RM. Conflicts of interest in the publication of science. JAMA 1991;266:266-267.

10. Koshland DE Jr. Conflict of interest policy. Science 1992;257:595-595.
11. Kassirer JP, Angell M. Financial conflicts of interest in biomedical research. N Engl J Med 1993;329:570-571.
12. Smith R. Conflict of interest and the BMJ. BMJ 1994;308:4-5.
13. Angell M, Kassirer JP. Editorials and conflicts of interest. N Engl J Med 1996;335:1055-1056.
14. The politics of disclosure. Lancet 1996;348(9028):627.
15. Campbell P. Declaration of financial interests. Nature 2001;412:751-751.
16. Davidoff F, DeAngelis CD, Drazen JM, et al. Sponsorship, authorship, and accountability. N Engl J Med 2001;345:825-826.
17. Information for Authors. Crit Care Resusc 2002;4:326-328.
18. Piel G. The age of science: what scientists learned in the 20th century. New York: Basic Books, 2001:38-39.
19. Collier J, Iheanacho I. The pharmaceutical industry as an informant. Lancet 2002;360(9343):1405-1409.
20. Rochon PA, Gurwitz JH, Simms RW, et al. A study of manufacturer-supported trials of nonsteroidal anti-inflammatory drugs in the treatment of arthritis. Arch Intern Med 1994;154:157-163.
21. Montaner JS, O'Shaughnessy MV, Schechter MT. Industry-sponsored clinical research: a double-edged sword. Lancet 2001;358(9296):1893-1895.
22. Worthley LIG. Please read the fine print. Criti Care Resusc 2001;3:209-210.
23. Cullen DJ. Ghostwriting in scientific anesthesia journals. Anesthesiology 1997;87:195-196.
24. Rennie D, Flanagin A. Authorship! Authorship! Guests, ghosts, grafters, and the two-sided coin. JAMA 1994;271:469-471.
25. Relman AS. Separating continuing medical education from pharmaceutical marketing. JAMA 2001;285:2009-2012.

The Lancet is my hero; I shall not want

"Courage is what it takes to stand up and speak; courage is also what it takes to sit down and listen."
Winston Churchill

In what must be one of the most piercing medical editorials in recent times and with a crusading style reminiscent of Ralph Nader, the Lancet (October 25th 2003) condemned the CEO of AstraZeneca (Tom McKillop) for his marketing approach to rosuvastatin in attempting to muscle in on the billion dollar 'statin' market.[1]

What makes the editorial even more interesting is the fact that the Lancet has only two drug company advertisements in their October 25th 2003 issue, with AstraZeneca being one of the companies advertising Nexium® (esomeprazole) on the back page of the journal. This advertisement also appears on the back page of all previous issues of the Lancet for the year 2003. So it is (was?) quite a 'money-spinner' for the journal.

Following the publishing of the editorial, the initial conversation between Tom McKillop and Richard Horton (editor of the Lancet) must have been fairly robust. The formal reply to the editorial (November 1st 2003) only barely hides the pique felt by the AstraZeneca CEO when he declares his position in the 'statin wars' by saying "I deplore the fact that a respected scientific journal such as the Lancet should make such an outrageous critique of a serious, well studied, and important medicine."[2]

This highlights once again the relationship between the pharmaceutical industry and the medical profession. Information for physicians should be completely independent and devoid of 'spin'. However, in a multi-billion dollar market, drug companies will go to almost any length in an attempt to improve shareholder equity,[3,4] a position that many retirees may agree with when reviewing their superannuation portfolios, but perhaps not when considering their own health. The statement by the AstraZeneca CEO that "it is unthinkable that we should desist from our efforts to make this medicine [rosuvastatin] more widely available to physicians and patients" further indicates his strength of feeling when promoting his company's product.[2]

At a meeting of the International Committee of Medical Journal Editors, a statement supporting editorial freedom was prepared and promulgated.[5] While editorial freedom for a medical journal may be beyond question, it may come at a financial cost. Nevertheless, if a journal prefers not to compromise its fiscal position by confronting important scientific issues, it does so at the risk of becoming irrelevant.

REFERENCES
1. Editorial. The statin wars: why AstraZeneca must retreat. Lancet 2003;362(9393):1341.
2. McKillop T. The statin wars. Lancet 2003;362(9394):1498.
3. Bodenheimer T. Uneasy alliance: clinical investigators and the pharmaceutical industry. N Engl J Med 2000;342:1539-1544.
4. Thomas PS, Tan KS, Yates DH. Sponsorship, authorship, and accountability. Lancet 2002;359(9303):351.
5. Editorial freedom: A Statement by the International Committee of Medical Journal Editors. Lancet 1988;2(8619):1089.

Are drug companies using or abusing science?

"Since we can never know anything for sure, it is simply not worth searching for certainty; but it is well worth searching for truth; and we do this chiefly by searching for mistakes, so that we can to correct them."
Karl Popper

"If Xigris is not used in one of our severely septic patients and they die, I would recommend to the relatives that they sue," said one of the intensivists.

We had just been discussing the recent PROWESS (recombinant human activated PROtein C Worldwide Evaluation in Severe Sepsis) trial[1] at our weekly journal club meeting. The trial was a prospective, randomised, placebo-controlled multicenter study of 1690 patients with severe sepsis (i.e. systemic inflammation and one or more organ failures) who received either the Eli Lilly drug, Xigris® (i.e. drotrecogin alfa activated – a drug with anti-inflammatory and anticoagulant activities) or placebo. As the drug was associated with an increased risk of bleeding, patients who had trauma or had undergone recent surgery, had a stroke within the previous 3 months, platelet count of < 30,000, chronic liver disease or anticoagulation with heparin or warfarin, were excluded.

The result: Xigris® was associated with a reduction in the 28 day mortality from 30.83% to 24.72% (i.e. 1 additional life saved for every 16 patients treated).[1] "This is undisputable evidence!" said the intensivist. A press release from Eli Lilly at the time of the 15th Annual Congress of the European Society of Intensive Care Medicine, Barcelona 2002, added that they had 'data showing treatment with Xigris® resulted in a 22 percent reduction in the relative risk of death in sicker severe sepsis patients with two or more organ dysfunctions', and that 'Xigris demonstrated an even higher reduction in the relative risk of death than in the full landmark PROWESS trial.'

L. I. G. Worthley

However, some of the intensive care specialists at the meeting were less than convinced. Controversy had already surrounded the trial. For example, in the latter half of the study the entry criteria changed. It shifted the population towards patients with less severe underlying disease and more acute infectious illness. A different cell line for the production of Xigris® was used, and 20 research sites were removed and 45 new sites were added.[2,3] As the drug did not improve survival in patients enrolled before these modifications,[2,4] clearly another study was needed. Surely one cannot change the rules half way through the trial and then report the results as if it were a single study?

Drug companies have provided millions of dollars towards research and development and have introduced many important agents for a wide range of diseases. However, the marketing of their 'groundbreaking' drugs can be vigorous and relentless, using techniques of spin, concealment and distortion and organising promotions that can barely be called continuing medical education meetings. In 2001 an estimated 35 billion dollars were spent by the pharmaceutical industry on these activities.[5]

While companies opine that drugs are expensive because they are costly to develop and produce, the fact is they spend more than twice as much on marketing and administration than they do on research and development. In the 5 years from 1998 to 2002, 415 new drugs were approved by the Food and Drug Administration (FDA), of which only 14% were truly innovative. A further 9% were old drugs that had been changed in some way that made them, in the FDA's view, significant improvements. And the remaining 77% were me-too drugs (e.g. a molecule would be changed to the older drug to provide 20 years of patient rights to counter the out of patent older drug which was no longer profitable). These me-to drugs were classified by the FDA as being no better than drugs already on the market to treat the same condition.[6] The reason for the FDA approval? The new drugs only have to be shown to be more effective than a placebo and not the currently used drug. So the new drug may be just as effective or even less effective than the standard drug.

The most notable misrepresentations by drug companies have been:
a. Vioxx® study which reported a significant reduction in upper gastrointestinal bleeding, but tended to obscure the doubling of the risk of heart attacks and strokes in the data presented to the FDA.[7] In a press release on 4 Nov 2004, the FDA estimated that Vioxx® may have contributed to 27,785 heart attacks and sudden cardiac deaths between 1999 and 2003.[8] During that period Vioxx® generated about $2.5 billion in yearly sales for the drug company Merck.

Merck withdrew Vioxx® from the market on September 2004 and one wonders whether the company only considered withdrawing the drug when profits from the sale of the drug were less than the payments for lawsuits from the deaths it caused.

b. Celebrex® study which reported a lower rate of serious gastrointestinal bleeding than either ibuprofen or diclofenac using the first 6 months of data. However, using the first 12 months of data, Celebrex® had a higher rate of serious gastrointestinal bleeding than either ibuprofen or diclofenac.[9]

Recently massive fines have been metered out to drug companies for marketing 'indiscretions'. For example: GlaxoSmithKline (GSK) will pay $3bn (£1.9bn) in the largest healthcare fraud settlement in US history. The drug giant was guilty in illegally promoting the antidepressants Paxil® and Wellbutrin® for unapproved uses (i.e. off-label marketing) including treatment of children and adolescents, and failing to report safety data about a diabetes drug Avandia® to the FDA. It also agreed to resolve civil liability for promoting the asthma drug Advair® and two lesser-known drugs for unapproved uses. In addition, GSK was found guilty of paying kickbacks to doctors.[10]

Pfizer has agreed to pay the federal government $60 million to settle allegations that its employees bribed doctors and other foreign officials in Europe and Asia to win business and boost sales. The charges against Pfizer were brought under the Foreign Corrupt Practices Act, which bars publicly traded companies from bribing officials in other countries to get or retain business. In 2011 Johnson and Johnson agreed to pay $70 million to settle civil and criminal charges of bribery brought by the Department of Justice.[11]

Returning to the Xigris® saga, a significant adverse effect on survival in critically ill patients with Xigris® at 1-year follow-up was reported in 2004.[12] The ADDRESS trial (a randomised study reviewing the effects of Xigris® on survival in patients with severe sepsis and critical illness) was terminated in 2005 after enrolment of 2000 of an anticipated 11000 patients, due to concerns that it may have been harmful.[13,14] Notwithstanding these negative studies, by late 2005 Eli Lilly had recorded sales of $214.6 million despite concerns about its efficacy.[15] In 2011 Eli Lilly recorded Xigris® sales of $100 million.[16] Finally, another trial (the PROWESS-SHOCK trial) was launched to answer concerns about the efficacy of the drug in patients who were most likely to be treated with Xigris® (e.g. patients in septic shock).[17] On 25 October 2011, Eli Lilly announced that it was withdrawing Xigris® from the market in response to the negative results of this trial.[18,19]

Xigris® was used twice in our intensive care unit following the weekly meeting in 2002. No one was sued.

REFERENCES
1. Bernard GR, Vincent J-L, Laterre P-F, LaRosa SP, Dhainaut J-F, Lopez-Rodriguez A, et al, for the Recombinant Human Activated Protein C Worldwide Evaluation in Severe Sepsis (PROWESS) Study Group. Efficacy and safety of recombinant human activated protein C for severe sepsis. N Engl J Med 2001;344:699-709.
2. Warren HS, Suffredini AF, Eichacker PQ, Munford RS. Risks and benefits of activated protein C treatment for severe sepsis. N Engl J Med 2002;347:1027-1030.
3. Wenzel RP. Treating sepsis. N Engl J Med 2002;347:966-967.
4. Siegel JP. Assessing the use of activated protein C in the treatment of severe sepsis. N Engl J Med 2002;347:1030-1034.

5. Angell M. The truth about the drug companies. How they deceive us and what to do about it. New York: Random House Trade Paperbacks, 2005; p136
6. Ibid. p75
7. Abramson J. Overdo$ed America. New York: Harper Perennial, 2004. p33-36.
8. FDA estimates Vioxx caused 27,785 deaths http://www.consumeraffairs.com/news04/vioxx_estimates.html (accessed April 2012)
9. Abramson J. Overdo$ed America. New York: Harper Perennial, 2004. p 29-31.
10. www.bbc.co.uk/news/world-us-canada-18673220 (accessed August 2012)
11. www.cbsnews.com/8301-501367_162-57488456/pfizer-pays-$60-million-to-settle-bribery-charges (accessed August 2012)
12. Angus DC, Laterre P-F, Helterbrand J, Ely W, Ball DE, Garg R, et al, for the PROWESS Investigators. The effect of drotrecogin alfa (activated) on long-term survival after severe sepsis. Crit Care Med 2004;32:2199-2206.
13. Deans KJ, Mineci PC, Eichacker PQ, Natanson C. The efficacy of drotrecogin alfa depends on severity of illness. Crit Care Med 2004;32:2347.
14. Abraham E, Laterre P-F, Garg R, Levy H, Talwar D, Trzaskoma BL, et al, for the Administration of Drotrecogin Alfa (Activated) in Early Stage Severe Sepsis (ADDRESS) Study Group. Drotrecogin alfa (Activated) for adults with severe sepsis and low risk of death. N Engl J Med 2005;353:1332-1341.
15. Eichacker PQ, Natanson C, Danner RL. Surviving sepsis – practice guidelines, marketing campaigns, and Eli Lilly. N Engl J Med 2006;355:1640-1642.
16. Bellomo R, Lipcsey M. Xigris 2011: déjà vu all over again? Crit Care Resusc 2011;13:211-212.
17. Finfer S, Ranieri VM, Thompson BT, Barie PS, Dhainaut JF, Douglas IS, et al. Design, conduct, analysis and reporting of a

multi-national placebo-controlled trial of activated protein C for persistent septic shock. Intensive Care Med 2008;34:1935-1947.
18. Lilly Announces Withdrawal of Xigris® Following Recent Clinical Trial Results http://www.prnewswire.com/news-releases/lilly-announces-withdrawal-of-xigris-following-recent-clinical-trial-results-132519063.html (accessed March 2012)
19. Ranieri VM, Thompson BT, Barie PS, Dhainaut J-F, Douglas IS, Finfer S, et al, for the PROWESS-SHOCK Study Group. Drotrecogin alfa (activated) in adults with septic shock. N Engl J Med 2012;366:2055-2064.

Section 5. Reflections

Do public hospital CEO's have a sense of humour?

"It ain't so much the things we don't know that get us into trouble. It's the things we know that just ain't so."
Artemus Ward

I guess I just don't like unproven and potentially harmful therapy. Once I asked the first question about a suspect medical practice I could not stop. And so it was in the case of the new hyperbaric chamber that arrived at our hospital along with a team of disciples who advanced its therapeutic powers for a whole range of conditions including the management of burns. As far as I could determine, apart from decompression sickness and air embolism, hyperbaric oxygen had no evidence-based therapeutic indication.

I used to give lectures on 'advances in acute medical therapy' and was often asked "what about hyperbaric oxygen?" Initially I would say that apart from decompression sickness and air embolism I knew of no evidence-based indication. However, I soon began to reply that I had written a short précis on the indications for hyperbaric oxygen (HBO) – it consisted of one sheet of blank A4 paper. For the comprehensive text it was two sheets of blank A4 paper.

As a recently appointed department head of anaesthesia and intensive care at the RAH was one of the HBO enthusiasts, it perhaps was not a smart thing for me to do to continue to challenge his belief. Nevertheless, an article appeared in a prominent international medical journal that completely supported my opinion concerning the absence of therapeutic indications for HBO.[1] I wrote a letter to the senior author of the paper (Dr. E. Robin) agreeing with his analysis, to find six months later that he included part of my letter in his reply to the

193

L. I. G. Worthley

RAH department's criticism of his article, both of which were published in the correspondence section of the journal.[2,3] He wrote, "I have received a letter from one of your colleagues at the Royal Adelaide Hospital who describes your treatment of burns patients and the activities of your group in general as follows: 'The Royal Adelaide Hospital has just acquired a Hyperbaric Unit along with a group of zealous individuals who operate this facility. Many of the diseases you mentioned (which we once felt that we had under reasonable control) are now referred almost routinely to the HBO unit for treatment. To refuse to do so has even been suggested to us that we may be liable for malpractice. What I find interesting is that if the patient improves it is always due to the HBO therapy, whereas if the patient gets worse then it is because we have not referred the patient early enough for HBO therapy'". Dr. Robin then added "this is hardly the description of an unbiased, rational, trustworthy group of physicians" – mercilessly humiliating, at an international level, our department head and five other doctors.

Following this episode, while I may have had tenure at the RAH, I knew it was going to be uphill from here.

Initially, for my sins, I was asked by the head of the department to do some anaesthetic lists. I informed him, however, that I was unable to do so as I was not registered as an anaesthetist, had not performed an anaesthetic for the past 15 or so years, and had been appointed specifically as a specialist in intensive care medicine at the hospital. Next I was asked to appear before the chief executive officer.

The chief executive officer, a quietly spoken man, required me to wait outside his office until his secretary was asked to usher me in. He sat low behind his desk and, without our usual pleasantries, read from a prepared statement informing me that due to the hospital's budget constraints we had to be involved in multi-skilling of staff, and that my duties had been broadened to include anaesthetic lists.

"But I am not registered," I said.

"You will need to be retrained," he stated.

"Terrific!" I said, "if the hospital was intending to embrace multi-skilling and retraining I want to do brain surgery!"

He replied (sotto voce), "don't be funny Tub, we are serious in our approach across all specialties."

"Frogshit!" I thought, as I was the only person in the whole hospital let alone the department of anaesthesia and intensive care who was required to be retrained.

"So what will you be retrained as?" I asked him, poker-faced.

His lower neck reddened. "Tub..." he began.

Suddenly his phone rang. He held his hand up to halt any further discussion and picked up the receiver.

"Hello." He then held his hand over the mouthpiece, "it's the Premier of South Australia, I will have to speak to you later." I thought about giving him a clever reply but fortunately didn't, because thankfully our problems ultimately resolved and the 'serious approach across all specialties to multi-skilling' at the hospital was abandoned.

Why do public hospital administrators make life so difficult? Is it because they have no sense of humour, or because they find it difficult to deal with difficult people like me? Private hospital administrators seem to be a different species. They are pleasant and willing to work toward a common goal of providing the best facilities for the patients and best working environment for their staff. Whenever there was a problem I could phone them at any time and work the issue out without being required to sit outside their office waiting to be summoned.

At any meeting I had with public hospital administrative staff, I would get clichés, not solutions: "my hands are tied", "I would like to help", "I'm between a rock and a hard place" and "this hurts me more than it does you." If the Minister of Health and the media were not bothering them concerning, for example, some patient who died unattended in the emergency department, then they were happy. The public hospital would just grind on. Perhaps that's the style of management in any public service. If you keep your head down and don't ask embarrassing questions, everything will be fine; but if you question the authorities, it's very likely the authorities will question you.

REFERENCES
1. Gabb G, Robin ED. Hyperbaric oxygen. A therapy in search of diseases. Chest 1987;92:1074-1082.
2. Runciman WB, Gorman DF, Webb RK, Russell WJ, Gilligan JE, Parsons DW. Letters to the editor. Chest 1988;671-672.
3. Robin ED. Letters to the editor. Chest 1988;94:672-673.

Return to my *Alma Mater*

"... *I am not now*
That which I have been"
George Gordon Byron

I have been interested in postgraduate training of ICU specialists for most of my professional career; initially as a lecturer, then examiner and finally holding an annual postgraduate training course for those who wished to become intensivists. The postgraduate training course began in 1983 as a five day seminar at the Royal Adelaide Hospital (RAH) with the other major South Australian teaching hospitals taking a minor, but nonetheless important, role for a half or a full day of teaching. In 1992 both the course and I shifted to the Flinders Medical Centre. The Royal Adelaide Hospital was still involved, although for one day only, and for some years I did not oversee or attend their teaching sessions. However, eventually I went back to help with their clinical seminars.

Returning to the RAH after so many years was an interesting experience. While I immediately recognized the main corridors and hallways, with the untouched scratch marks on the walls at the level of the hospital barouches, many of the wards had changed. As I walked along each passage my mind conjured images and shadows of things that once were. Familiar echoes surrounded me then faded as I finally entered the ICU waiting room.

The ICU was now on a different floor. The ward clerk sat at her desk guarding the entrance to the unit. She was a recent employee and did not recognize me as a former intensive care specialist who had worked at the Royal Adelaide Hospital for 20 years. To her, I was just one of a number of concerned relatives, that milled around the ICU entrance, hungry for any information about their family, and anxious to get into the unit. The spirit and spectre of the ICU had changed. I was a stranger in a place that was my Alma Mater. "Suck it up and

197

move on," my daughter-in-law would say. "Nostalgia is an indulgence."

Suddenly one of the senior cardiologists, burst out of the intensive care unit entrance and spied me.

"Hello Tub. You're back then?"

"Err . . . not for good Peter, just back as an examiner for the ICU course."

"Ah, we need to get you back. We miss your obsession with radical therapy."

"Ha, diseases desperate grown . . . ." I mused and added "but I think that another Worthley at the RAH would be one too many for this hospital." (Two of my sons are employed as staff members at the RAH cardiology department.)

"That's not true. Another one would just round out the Trinity," he said, continuing to walk from the ICU. He gave me a kindly smile as he looked back, then waving his hand uttered "Ciao." He turned the corner and was gone.

"Ah . . ." I said trying to delay him from leaving so that I could have more time to chat, as I enjoyed our gentle banter. It made me feel welcome and indeed at home.

"Come in, Tub" was my next invitation. It was the ICU director pushing past the milling relatives. "You are right on time. You found the new unit then? Follow me."

"Thanks Rob," I said following close behind him.

We entered the unit after he swiped his key card over the electronic entry device, automatically swinging the doors open and allowing us to leave the throng of peering relatives behind.

"Some things have changed with the new unit," Rob explained "but the patients are still the same, perhaps older and sicker and, as always, more of them. The course registrants are a mixed bunch. Anyway we will let you make your own judgment."

He entered the lecture room and introduced me as "one of the 'early settlers' of Australasian ICU." He generously went on and on.

I responded by thanking him for his kind remarks saying,

"I can hardly wait to hear what I am about to say," (polite chuckle from the audience), and began my lecture.

I left some time later after finishing my session and having had a cup of tea and a biscuit with some of the course registrants and the ICU nursing staff. The latter I found more difficult to have a light conversation with than the course registrants. The generation gap had become wide. Perhaps I was distracted by their facial piercings.

I thought about my first visit back to the Royal Adelaide Hospital ICU for most of that evening. It was the hospital that had nurtured my interest in intensive care medicine for all of my formative years. My return made me realize that while I did not mind remembering my early years, I did not want to relive them. It helped me understand the beneficial effect of change. I had learnt so many different skills when I moved from the Royal Adelaide Hospital to the Flinders Medical Centre igniting once again my enthusiasm for acute medicine. Not so surprising really, because in any profession, to reinvigorate and move forward one needs to move on, and probably often.

On reflection

"And in the end, the love you get is equal to the love you give"
The Beatles

It was a strange time. I had just retired from my public clinical intensive care life along with the undergraduate and postgraduate teaching responsibilities and the journal of *Critical Care and Resuscitation* editorial duties. However I was still involved in clinical practice at three private hospital intensive care units, and enjoyed my extra time with patients and their relatives. I could now converse with them without thinking about deadlines.

I began to settle back to a quieter lifestyle and was somewhat surprised to receive a note from the Joint Faculty of Intensive Care Medicine – the Australasian training and accrediting body for intensivists – recommending me for the Joint Faculty medal. As I was required to deliver a 15 minute address before I received the award at the Faculty's annual scientific meeting dinner in Melbourne in June 2006, I decided to 'reflect and predict' the future of intensive care medical practice. At that meeting I opined:

"I will use this occasion to briefly reflect on my professional life, to look forward and view what perhaps could be the future for intensive care medicine, and to highlight the importance of teaching, research and writing in the development of our discipline. My experience is modest, but it may be of interest to those of you who are just embarking on your career as an intensivist. Over the past 35 years, there have been numerous changes in bedside diagnostic and therapeutic techniques to benefit the critically ill patient. There have also been changes to the ICU admission criteria. The patients are now older, sicker, and have many comorbid conditions. To accommodate this group, intensive care units have had to increase their bed numbers and expand their services. Units have quadrupled in size and are often required to offer medical emergency teams, venous access and parenteral nutrition services to other inpatients, and retrieval, mechanical ventilation and parenteral nutrition services to many outpatients. Patients can now be suspended physiologically for weeks, using modern cardiovascular, respiratory and renal support techniques. Withdrawal of therapy has now become an accepted part of our clinical practice, with relatives and friends often struggling to understand the diagnosis of futility. Where are we heading – particularly with an ageing population, a greater expectation from the public (and our medical colleagues) as to the benefits of ICUs, and as the subspecialties of surgery and medicine (even palliative care medicine) increasingly want our units to manage their patients? Will the major teaching hospital simply become one large intensive care unit, with all patients monitored and measured, and all non-critically ill patients managed at home or in dedicated medical hotels, with telemetry keeping the clinician in touch with their progress? Hospitals as intensive care units, and intensivists as hospitalists?

Will these large ICUs become more 'open' and administered by nurses, with intensivists becoming resuscitationists, and treatment being largely protocolised or managed by the home team? Goodness knows. However, if a community believes that their hospitals should have 20, 40 or 60 ICU beds (or even 1000 ICU beds) to manage acutely ill patients, then medical, as well as nursing numbers, must be commensurate to meet this need, otherwise the unit becomes dysfunctional. A culture of inertia develops, the unit is always full, and 'we have no beds' is the constant refrain. For patients who do get admitted to the ICU, so long as they have 'normal' physiological values (e.g. blood pressure, pulse, arterial PaO_2 and pH), they remain deeply sedated, mechanically ventilated and on inotropic support, until a diagnosis of 'futility' is made, and withdrawal of therapy is seriously considered. Patient care is substandard, the medical team is without enthusiasm, there is no time for formal teaching or research, and there is a high turnover of proficient staff, with those who are without skill tending to remain. For the sake of future critically ill patients, intensive care units must remain with a 'closed' format, and public teaching hospitals must allocate no more than 12 ICU beds per intensivist, with at least one advanced intensive care trainee and four primary trainees for the same number of beds. This means that the matter of a diminishing number of doctors being attracted to our discipline must be addressed urgently. To increase our numbers we need more units with directors generating an atmosphere of excitement and fun, while providing vibrant and active teaching and research programs.

This requires intelligent and creative public hospital chairs, boards of directors and CEOs, employing talented intensivists and allowing them a free hand. As the cost of wanting to maintain life is soaring, a large amount of additional money for the public system will also be required. However, as with any enterprise, unless competent administrative staff are employed, these funds will be wasted, as an able ICU director cannot be effective in the face of poor hospital management.

Over the past 35 years, therapeutic agents to treat acutely ill patients have come and gone. Aprotinin for pancreatitis, thiopentone for cerebral resuscitation, sodium bicarbonate for cardiac arrest, dopamine for acute renal failure (all once 'mandatory' treatments) have now largely disappeared. Over the same period, Australasian intensive care research and education have been advancing. Clinical research has been put on a solid platform, largely due to the efforts of the Australian and New Zealand Intensive Care Society's clinical trials group, while annual educational courses in South Australia, Queensland, New South Wales and Victoria, supplementing the Joint Faculty accreditation process, have made the clinical training of Australasian intensivists second to none.

Yet, in spite of these advances, the question remained, "What about the written word?" To our new graduates I would say this: there is nothing like writing to force you to get your thoughts straight. It sharpens the intellect like no other communication, as you place your thoughts in the public arena for scrutiny and critique. The experience may be brutal, but is rewarding and necessary if you wish to communicate globally. Concerning the Australasian intensive care medical scene: as I aged, the more intensely I believed that we needed our own journal to encourage our trainees to write and submit articles to a relevant publication. While some believed that we were serviced effectively by journals that were currently available, others did not. Undaunted, in March 1999 and heading into a stiff headwind of criticism, a quarterly entitled *Critical Care and Resuscitation* was

Inside God's Shed

published. However, I wasn't alone in this venture and must acknowledge many people: Andrew Holt, Andrew Bersten, Rinaldo Bellomo, Bala Venkatesh, John Morgan, Neil Matthews, Jamie Cooper, John Myburgh and John Moran, among others, contributed without hesitation to this novice publication. Indeed, it was hard to stop John Moran whenever I asked him to submit a statistical piece, and, bless their hearts, Rinaldo Bellomo and John Morgan would always write the antithesis to every piece I presented on strong ions. Geoff Parkin even submitted a piece pertaining to the mean systemic pressure (a notion which he firmly believes is the 'big bang' theory of the circulation). Neil Matthews has always been supportive and, as Dean of the Joint Faculty of Intensive Care Medicine, was instrumental in making *Critical Care and Resuscitation* the journal of the Joint Faculty, commencing from March 2004. He also suggested that Vernon van Heerden would be an ideal editor to shepherd the publication through its next phase. Both ideas have not only served the journal well, but have enhanced its standing. The journal is now Medline indexed. I must also thank Paul Glover who, from the Royal Victoria Hospital in Belfast, tirelessly reviewed with me most of the journal's manuscripts during the first 6 years. Thank goodness for email.

Finally, I must thank my wife Janice. When she first realized that I was considering writing, editing, publishing, posting and soliciting manuscripts and subscriptions for a new journal, she was not all that enthused and asked me "Why?" I think I said, "Life is a great big canvas; throw all the paint on it you can", which I don't think helped, as she responded, "Well make sure that you don't use any of my paint and don't splash my canvas." It wasn't her dream. Nevertheless, during the first 6 years of the Journal's life, she helped enormously as she managed the advertisements and merchant banking and allowed our kitchen table to be the Journal's 'canvas'. Indeed, I think that she was even a little sad when we finally handed all this over to the Joint Faculty secretariat.

Incidentally, during the past year or so, while I have spent more time at home quietly and at leisure, I have probably not warmed as much to Janice's ideas of gardening, tidying the shed, pruning roses or cleaning gutters as I should have. So much so that, when I told her I

203

was about receive the Joint Faculty award of a medal, she said, "What exactly does this award do?" I replied, "Well it doesn't do anything." She shrugged and said, "Then they are giving it to the right person!"

I have had a fortunate and enjoyable professional life and have met many amazing people along the way: the fun and fellowship I had with the first ANZICS executive, with people like Bob Wright, Geoff Clarke and Malcolm Fisher making decisions for the Society with little reference to anyone; the arguments we had with the Faculty of Anaesthetists and the College of Physicians during the development of the inaugural ICU diplomas; the ease with which we were able to undertake many of our early clinical studies before ethics committees were mandatory; the eagerness and enthusiasm of trainees when they saw their first article in print; the ICU nursing staff, for whom I have enormous respect, and their tolerance of my occasional acidic remark; and finally the sharing of both joy and grief with critically ill patients and their relatives. I have loved it all."

Acknowledgements

I would like to thank my wife Janice for her unconditional love and support. To our sons Stephen, Matthew and Daniel and our grandchildren: William, Phoebe, Harry, Thomas, Charlotte, Beth, James and Chloe, thank you for sharing with us your endless enthusiasm and passion for life.

I am indebted to Dr. Paul Glover whose editorial skills throughout my years of publishing the journal *Critical Care and Resuscitation* compelled me to impose upon his good nature once again to correct my spelling and syntax errors in this book.

I must also thank the many doctors and nurses who have tolerated my numerous faults and frailties during my career as an intensivist. And to the many patients and their relatives who have allowed me to enter their lives and share their journeys with me, I hope that I have been helpful.

About the Author

Dr. Lindsay Ian Grant Worthley worked as an intensive care medical specialist at the Royal Adelaide Hospital intensive care unit (ICU) for 20 years (1971-1991) and at the Flinders Medical Centre ICU for 16 years (1991-2007). He resigned from public intensive care practice in 2007 and spent 2 years as an intensivist at three of Adelaide's private hospitals. He retired from clinical intensive care practice in 2009 although he still teaches postgraduate students. He has published over 130 indexed scientific articles and books that include:

- Worthley LIG. Synopsis of Intensive Care Medicine. London: Churchill Livingstone, 1994
- Worthley LIG. Handbook of Emergency Laboratory Tests. New York: Churchill Livingstone, 1996.
- Worthley LIG. Clinical examination of the critically ill patient, 3rd Ed. Melbourne: The Australasian Academy of Critical Care Medicine, 2006.

He will be remembered largely as a postgraduate teacher in intensive care medicine, establishing and supervising the Adelaide postgraduate intensive care medicine course from 1983 – 2005. His research interests include, oxygen uptake, fluid, electrolyte and acid-base abnormalities in the critically ill patient, total parenteral nutrition in hospital and home patients and percutaneous tracheostomy.

He is married to Janice and has 3 sons and 8 grandchildren, all of whom he loves dearly. In 2010 he was appointed as a Member in the General Division of the Order of Australia (AM) for 'Service to medical education, particularly in the area of intensive care medicine, as a clinician, mentor and educator, and through contributions to professional associations'.

Email: lindsaywrty@gmail.com

Index

ABBA, 61
abdominal
  abscess, 17
  aortic aneurysm, 71
  binder, 48
  wound, 46
Accident and Emergency
  consultant, 9
  department, 9
  resident, 69
acetone, 10
acetylene, 29
acid-base
  Stewart approach, 158
  strong ion difference, 158
acidosis
  metabolic, 45, 66
Actrapid®
  treatment of diltiazem overdose, 52
acupuncture, 100
ADDRESS trial, 190
adhesions
  multiple bowel, 44
adrenaline, 6, 9
adverse events
  calculated risk, 112
  classification, 112
  definition, 110
  in critically ill patients, 111
  preventable, 112
  unpreventable, 112
albumin
  intravenous, 160
  production, 160
  properties, 160
  synthesis, 161
allergic reaction, 47

Alma Mater, 197
Alternative therapy, 99
Ambu™ bag, 9
amiodarone, 9, 57, 125
amlodipine, 51, 57
anaesthesia
  general, 12
anaesthesia and intensive care, 195
analbuminaemia, 161
analgesia
  local, 12
  patient controlled, 84
Apollo mission, 114
appendicectomy, 17
  retrocaecal, 44
Aprotinin, 202
arterial blood
  gas, 30
asthma
  treatment
    protocol, 65
AstraZeneca, 185
asystole, 9
atenolol, 27, 71
atrial fibrillation, 108
  chronic, 57
audit
  morbidity and mortality data, 110
  risk/benefit study, 110
Austin Moore prosthesis, 19
Australasian Association of Clinical
  Biochemists, 160
Australian and New Zealand
  Intensive Care Society, 182
  clinical trials group, 202
Avandia, 189

baby boomer, 93
bacterial peritonitis

209

Index

spontaneous, 163
Bacteroides spp, 45
base excess, 66
Bellomo, Rinaldo, 203
Bentall procedure, 80
Bersten, Andrew, 203
Berwick, Donald, 14
Bezwoda, W.R., 176
Birdsville, 29
Black, Douglas, 54
blood pressure
    maintenance, 149
blood transfusion, 6
bone atrophy, 36
bone marrow transplant, 109
Borg, Bjorn, 44
bowel
    fistula, 17
    gangrene, 46
    obstruction, 17
Bower, Albert, 3
brain
    damage, 39
    dead, 33
    death, 36, 134
Bread, 2
British Medical Journal, 181
budesonide, 65
Buffett, Warren, 26
Buist, Michael, 87
Byron, George Gordon, 197

calcium
    carbide, 29
    chloride, 10, 51
cancer
    breast, 176
        high-dose chemotherapy and bone marrow transplantation, 176
Cancer Council of Australia, 99
Cancer Society of America, 99
captopril, 26, 27

cardiac
    defibrillator, 5
    index, 27
    monitor, 5
cardiac arrest, 125
    asystolic, 47
    team, 125
cardiogenic shock, 72
cardiomyopathy, 125
cardiopulmonary
    bypass, 5
    resuscitation, 9, 125
        'slow code', 135
cardioversion, 1
    anticoagulation, 108
care
    quality of, 113
Carlon, G. C., 3
carnitine deficiency, 47
Carroll, Lewis, 68
carvedilol, 58
Celebrex, 189
central venous catheter, 12, 14
    infection
        checklist, 37
cerebral oedema, 39
checklists, 35
    anaesthetic, 36
    nursing, 36
    postgraduate examination, 36
    surgical, 36
chlorpromazine, 20
church
    Assemblies of God, 49
Churchill, Winston, 9, 132, 147, 175, 185
Ciardi, John, 144
cimetidine
    intravenous, 47
cirrhosis, 48
Clarke, Geoff, 204
clinical
    examination, 149

Index

judgement, 42
Clostridium perfringens, 45
Cochrane Collaboration, 100, 164
Cochrane Library, 145
coffee break, 119
College of Intensive Care Medicine of Australia and New Zealand, 156
College of Physicians, 204
colloidal silver
   inhalation, 95
coma, 46
comfort care, 135
comfort care only, 88
complementary and alternative medical therapies, 98
conflict of interest
   definition, 181
Confucius, 57
consultation
   medical, 42
Coolidge, Calvin, 44
Cooper, Jamie, 203
copper wrist bracelet, 101
coronary artery
   bypass graft, 23
coronary care unit, 126
C-reactive protein, 27
Critical Care and Resuscitation, 202
critical illness polyneuropathy, 47
Crowfoot, Betsy, 174
Curtin, Leah, 138
cytokines
   inflammatory, 161

Da Vinci, Leonardo, 154
Dalrymple, Theodore, 108
Danderfield, Rodney, 39
Danish poliomyelitis epidemic, 3
Darwin, Charles, 1
DDAVP®, 6
death
   prediction of time to die, 135
   prolongation, 133
decerebrate, 33
delirium tremens, 19
dementia, 79
Department of Justice, 190
Devil's Claw, 101
dexamethasone
   intravenous, 41
diabetes
   type 1, 11
   type 2, 121
dialysis, 45, 46
Dickens, Charles, 16
Dickinson, Emily, 129
diclofenac, 189
digoxin, 27, 57
diltiazem
   overdose, 51
do not resuscitate, 88
Doe, John, 9
dopamine, 202
drug companies
   marketing, 188
Dudrick, Stanley, 14

E. coli, 45
EACA, 6
echocardiograph
   transthoracic, 27
editorial freedom, 175
Einstein, Albert, 176
Eli Lilly, 187
embolism
   pulmonary, 36
Emerson, Ralph Waldo, 65
emphysema
   terminal, 132
encephalopathy, 48
end of life, 131
   management of, 131
esomeprazole, 185
European Society of Intensive Care Medicine, 187

Index

evidence-based medicine, 96, 145
exfolative dermatitis, 47
external cardiac massage, 9, 10

Faculty of Anaesthetists, 204
fee for service, 61
    gap, 62
    no gap, 62
femur
    fractured neck of, 19
Fisher, Malcolm, 204
fistula
    bowel, 46
    gastric, 46
    urethral, 47
flucloxacillin, 109
fluid balance
    negative, 147
Food and Drug Administration, 188
Foreign Corrupt Practices Act, 189
free radicals
    scavanged by albumin, 160
frusemide, 26, 30, 57
Fuldheim, Dorothy, 171
futility, 133

gas gangrene, 46
gastrectomy, 97
gastric erosions
    acute, 36
gastric stress ulcers, 46
Gelofusine, 71, 148
generation X, 93
ghost-writing, 182
Glasgow coma score, 39
GlaxoSmithKline, 189
Glover, Paul, 203
goat's milk, 95
gratuity, 8
grieving
    stages of, 129
GTN, 30
guardian, 79

guidelines, 35
    definition, 114
    limitations, 114

haemodynamic measurements
    zero referencing, 111
hand washing
    poor compliance, 111
Harrison, George., 141
Hartmann's solution, 71
Hawke, Neil, 44
Hawthorn, 101
head injury
    closed, 39
    severe, 39
health services
    access to, 139
heart failure
    systolic, 58
heparin
    subcutaneous, 36
hepatitis
    ischaemic, 27
    septic, 27
hepatitis B, 48
hepatitis C, 48
herbalism, 95
hernia
    incisional, 44
high dependency unit, 82
Hippocrates, 97, 141
Holt, Andrew, 203
homeopathy, 95
Horse chestnut, 101
Horton, Richard, 185
Hospice
    Mary Potter, 48
Hospital
    administrators, 195
    appointment, 151
    Blegdam, 3
    Bundaberg Base, 18
    Burnley General, 44

Index

Flinders Medical Centre, 197
Flinders Private, 62
Los Angeles County General, 3
Modbury, 44
Queen Elizabeth, 130
Royal Adelaide, vii, 197
Royal Victoria, 203
House of God, 30
Hutchison, Robert, 125, 141
hydrochloric acid
    intracatheter, 47
hydrocortisone
    intravenous for asthma, 65
hydrogen ion
    metabolism, 159
hyperbaric oxygen, 193
hyperglycaemia, 36
hyperkalaemia, 10
hyperventilation, 41, 66
hypoalbuminaemia, 161
    mortality, 161
hypokalaemia, 20
hypotension
    postural, 47

Ibsen, Bjorn, 3
ibuprofen, 189
induced coma, 54
informed consent, 113
inotropic agents, 46
insulin
    infusion, 10
    sliding scale, 36
insulin and glucose
    treatment of calcium channel
        blockers, 52
intensive care
    Adelaide postgraduate training
        course, 197
    admission, 68
    admission and discharge
        responsibilities, 68
    anaesthesia and, 35

audit
    clinical care, 106
    death review, 106
changes
    admission criteria, 200
    diagnostic and therapeutic
        techniques, 200
closed unit, 201
    definition, 155
conscious state of patients in, 54
cost, 138
differences in clinical practice, 106
director, 178
directors, 202
educational courses, 202
entry block, 86
esprit de corps, 120
exit block, 86
future, 200
guidelines, 145
handover, 118
judgement of peers, 105
medicine
    development of, 4
    education and research
        program, 37
neonatal unit, 111
nurse, 91
nurses, 118
open unit, 201
    definition, 155
paediatric unit, 111
patient demographic, 138
practice
    improvement, 114
private, 61
referral, 121
short course, 151
specialist talk, 167
teacher, 146
teaching, 144
    algorithms, 145
trainee, 145

213

Index

unit
    admission and discharge policies, 155
    bed numbers, 201
    definition, 3
    function, 4
    indication for admission, 127
    staff, 3
    ward clerk, 197
intensivist
    Australian, 156
    cognitive development, 146
    patient numbers per, 201
intercessory prayer, 100
Intergovernmental Panel on Climate Change, 175
International Committee of Medical Journal Editors, 175, 181
intestinal obstruction, 44
intra aortic balloon pump, 5
intracranial pressure
    monitor, 39
intra-operative awareness, 54
ischaemic heart disease, 57, 121, 125

Johnson and Johnson, 190
Joint Faculty
    annual scientific meeting dinner, 200
    medal, 200
Joint Faculty of intensive care medicine, 200
journal
    Critical Care and Resuscitation, vii
Journal of the American Medical Association, 175

Kava extract, 101
ketoacidosis, 10
Kipling, Rudyard, 23
Kissinger, Henry, 158
Knaus, William, 4
Kocher, Gerhard, 118, 121
Kübler-Ross, Elizabeth, 129
Kurtz, Paul, 178
kwashiorkor, 162
kyphoscoliosis, 94

Lancet, 175, 185
laparotomy, 44, 45
    paramedian, 44
Lassen, Henry, 3
left bundle branch block, 30
life support, 123
    decision by patient, 133
    family decision, 134
    futility
        scoring systems, 134
    refusal of, 132, 134
    withdrawal, 152, 201
    withholding or withdrawing, 134
    management of, 131
lifter
    Jordan frame, 44
lignocaine, 9
Lipton, Bruce, 97
living will, 131
locked-in syndrome, 54
Luer lock, 20
Lundberg, George, 175
lung disease
    fibrotic, 130
lymphoma
    non-Hodgkin's, 23

Maimonides, 151
malnutrition, 36, 162
marasmus, 162
Marlex mesh, 44
marrow transplantation, 176
Matthew 7:1-2, 105
Matthews, Neil, 203
McEnroe, John, 44
McKillop, Tom, 185
McLuhan, Marshall, 79
mean systemic pressure, 203

Index

medical emergency team, 19, 85
    clinicians, 85
    indications for, 85
    meta-analyses of, 87
    problems with, 86
    prospective randomised controlled trial of, 87
Merck, 189
meropenem, 121
metaraminol, 71
midazolam, 12, 40, 147
miracle, 96
mitral regurgitation, 58
mitral valve disease, 57
Montgomery, Robert, 5
Moran, John, 203
Morgan, John, 203
morphine, 40, 122, 127, 147
    infusion, 83
    intravenous, 30
Mukherjee, Siddhartha, 176
multiple organ failure, 45
multi-skilling medical staff, 194
muscle wasting, 36
Myburgh, John, 203
myelodysplasia, 108

Nader, Ralph, 185
nasal cannulae, 31, 57
nasogastric suction, 44
naturopath, 94
Needham, Richard, 85
needle phobia, 12
negligence, 113
neurosurgeon, 40
Nexium, 185
nifedipine, 51
nocebo, 100
noradrenaline, 41, 148
not for CPR, 125
not for resuscitation, 108
nurse
    team leader, 32

undergraduate, 32
nutrition
    intravenous, 14
    parenteral, 14

ophthalmoscope
    prospective randomised controlled trial, 149
Osler, William, 141
ovarian carcinoma, 121
oxygen dependent, 132

pacemaker
    capture, 6
    temporary, 5
pain
    specialists, 82
    treatment of, 82
pain clinic
    acute, 82
    chronic, 82
Palaprin Forte, 101
palliation, 15, 124
palliative care, 153
palpating hand
    prospective randomised controlled trial, 149
pancuronium, 133
Paracelsus, 82
parenteral nutrition
    home, 48
Parkin, Geoff, 203
Patel, Jayant, 18
patient
    cardiac surgical, 5
    dying
        care of the, 34
    management, 42
    unconscious, 33
Paxil, 189
percussion hammer
    prospective randomised controlled trial, 149

Index

perinodopril, 57
Perutz, Max, 179
Pfizer, 189
pharmaceutical and instrument manufacturers, 180
pharmaceutical companies subsidiaries, 182
physical signs, 149
placebo, 99, 188
plasma
    fresh frozen, 6, 7, 46, 148
    oncotic pressure, 160
platelets, 6, 7, 46
Plato, 19
pneumonia
    aspiration, 126
    atypical, 36
policies
    development, 113
polio, 3
Popper, Karl, 178, 187
post hoc ergo propter hoc, 99
private practice, 61
pro-con debate, 158
    educational value, 159
propofol, 12
prospective randomised controlled trial, 98
    intravenous albumin, 163
    Xigris, 187
        withdrawn from the market, 190
prospective randomized controlled trial, 171
protocols, 35, 65
    development, 113
    limitations, 113
proton pump inhibitor, 36
PROWESS trial, 187
PROWESS-SHOCK trial, 190
Pseudomonas aeruginosa, 47, 96
psychotic, 21
PubMed, 167

pulmonary artery
    occlusion pressure, 27
    pressure, 27
pulmonary oedema, 57, 71, 125
    acute, 30
    fulminant, 72
    iatrogenic, 149

quartz crystal, 96
questions to ask your doctor, 25

radiation enteritis, 16
radiotherapy, 147
rectal carcinoma, 147
    bowel obstruction, 147
regression to the mean, 99
remuneration, 61
renal disease
    urinalysis, 142
renal failure, 28, 58, 126
    chronic, 48
research
    acute coronary syndrome, 172
        anticoagulant drugs, 172
        autonomic system blockers, 172
    conflict of interest, 181
    experimental drugs, 171
    fraud, 176
    human, 171
        informed consent, 171
        patient enrolment, 173
    peer review, 174
        conflict of interest, 174
respiratory distress, 66
respiratory failure, 122
    acute-on-chronic, 132
    post operative, 147
respiratory technicians, 118
Revans, Reg, 91
right heart catheter, 27
Rogers, Will, 12
rosuvastatin, 185

Index

Rudolph, Arthur, 114
Rushdie, Salman, 32

sacral bed sore, 47
salbutamol
    continuously nebulised, 65
    adverse effects, 66
saline
    heparinised, 20
school
    St Leonards primary, vii
scientific presentation, 178
    chairman, 178
scrotum, 47
second opinion, 23, 39
Seigworth, Gilbert, 71
Seldinger wire, 13
septicaemia, 45
    E. coli, 147
Shaw, George Bernard, 94
Shipman, Harold, 107
shock
    circulatory, 45
Simon, Paul, 110
sinus bradycardia, 47
sinus rhythm, 10, 30
sodium bicarbonate, 202
spironolactone, 26, 57
split skin graft, 46
sputum retention, 123
St John's wort, 100
ST segments, 71
Staphylococcus aureus
    methicillin resistant, 47
    septicaemia, 108
Staphylococcus epidermidis, 47
starvation
    adverse effects, 14
stethoscope, 127
    prospective randomised controlled trial, 149
stomach cancer
    treatment of, 97

stroke, 33
subcutaneous fat
    necrosis, 46
subdural haematoma, 108
    craniotomy, 109
superannuation portfolio, 185
suxamethonium, 133
swabs
    alcohol, 20
Swan Ganz catheter, 27, 57, 148
Syrus, Publilius, 51, 160

teaching
    at the bedside, 142
    post graduate, 142
    undergraduate, 141
tea-room, 119
terminally ill patient
    futility of treatment, 134
The Beatles, 200
thiopentone, 41, 132, 202
thoracic aortic aneurysm, 79
thrombosis
    deep vein, 36
tobacco industry, 182
tracheal stenosis
    treatment of, 47
tracheostomy, 4, 46, 130
transfusion, 46, 72
    adverse effects, 74
    indications for, 72
treatment
    active
        indications for, 132
    alternative, 15, 94
Tub, vii
tuning fork
    prospective randomised controlled trial, 149

ulcers
    limb, mouth and eye, 36
Uniting church minister, 16

217

Index

Valium®, 20
van Heerden, Vernon, 203
vasopressin, 51
vein
    subclavian, 12
Venkatesh, Bala, 203
ventilation
    mechanical, 46
    negative pressure tank, 4
    positive pressure, 3
ventilator
    mechanical, 5, 129
ventricular fibrillation, 6, 9
ventricular tachycardia, 6
verapamil, 51
Vioxx, 189
Virgil, 180
vitamin
    deficiency, 36

ward rounds
    intensive care unit, 118
Ward, Artemus, 193
warfarin, 57
Weed, Lawrence, 29
Wellbutrin, 189
White Willow Bark, 101
Wilde, Oscar, 167
Worthley, Daniel, 1
Worthley, Janice, 203
Worthley, Lindsay, 35
Worthley, Matthew, 1
Worthley, Stephen, 1
Wright, Bob, 204

Xigris, 182, 187
    controversy, 188
X-ray
    chest, 30

ziphisternum
    pseudomonas infection of, 48

www.ingramcontent.com/pod-product-compliance
Lightning Source LLC
Chambersburg PA
CBHW051752040426
42446CB00007B/328